||||| ||||| ||||| |||||

☑ P9-ECW-073

BIO
ER

WITHDRAWN

*Keeping
Track??
Place your
initials here-*

CARSON CITY LIBRARY

Ten Things
I Learned from
Bill Porter

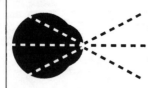This Large Print Book carries the
Seal of Approval of N.A.V.H.

Ten Things I Learned from
Bill Porter

Shelly Brady

Foreword by William H. Macy

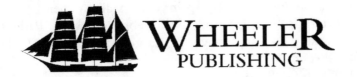
WHEELER
PUBLISHING

Copyright © 2002 by Shelly Brady

All rights reserved.

Published in 2002 by arrangement with New World Library.

Wheeler Large Print Softcover Series.

The text of this Large Print edition is unabridged.
Other aspects of the book may vary from the original edition.

Set in 16 pt. Plantin.

Printed in the United States on permanent paper.

Library of Congress Cataloging-in-Publication Data

Brady, Shelly, 1962–
    Ten things I learned from Bill Porter / Shelly Brady ;
foreword by William H. Macy. — Large print ed.
        p. cm.
    Originally published: Novato, Calif. : New World Library,
2002.
    ISBN 1-58724-351-2 (lg. print : sc : alk. paper)
    1. Porter, Bill — Health.   2. Cerebral palsy — Patients —
United States — Biography.   3. Large type books.   I. Title.
RC388.P67 B73 2002b
362.1′96836′0092—dc21
    [B]   2002033157

To

John,
Michelle, Katrina, Teressa,
Kevin, Erica, Emily,
Irene,
and Bill

Contents

Foreword by William H. Macy

If memory serves, I was on the phone yelling at the concierge about his tardiness in delivering a fax to my room as I put the videotape that my agent had sent me into the machine. It was the *20/20* piece about Bill Porter. The tape was only about eight minutes long, but by the end, I stood in my hotel room with the remote still in my hand, and wept like a baby. I wept for his dignity. I wept for his stoicism. And mostly I wept for his indomitable optimism. Later that day I showed the piece to my wife, and we held each other and wept. I then sent the tape to my writing partner Steven Schachter. He wept. Steven and I decided we had to try to write a screenplay about Bill Porter.

In the process of researching Bill's life, we saw another tape of one of Bill's motivational speeches, which he delivered with the help of his assistant, Shelly Brady. As we watched Shelly, I said to Steven, "This story just gets better and better. She's a babe."

A month or so later, Steven and I flew to Portland to meet Shelly and Bill. Shelly picked us up at the airport, or more correctly, she swept us up at the airport. She had the same indomitable spirit and optimism as Bill. Thirty-six hours later, both Steven and I were smitten. She and Bill had that rare relationship: synchronicity of thought, ease of being, mutual respect, and joy in each other's company. I explored the possibility of being adopted by them.

I think I should let Shelly tell her story now. It's a great story. And, as everyone in Hollywood knows, a great story is always better if it has a babe in it.

October 2001
Los Angeles, California

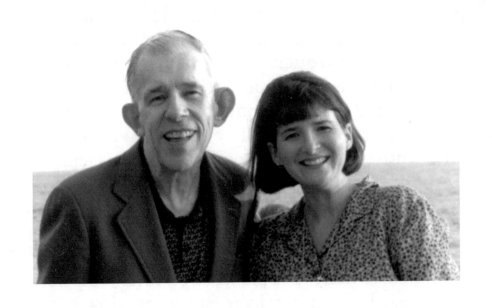

Introduction

Writers often speak of how their books wrote themselves, as if they were transcribing for a higher power. At times, while writing this book, I had a similar feeling. Each day before placing my fingers on the keyboard, I took a moment to ponder and pray, and then inspiration would come from above, leading me directly to Bill Porter himself. In spite of his cerebral palsy, he was able to overcome every obstacle he faced throughout his life and achieve all of his goals. Any momentary inability I had committing words to paper paled in comparison to the incredible challenges that Bill has met during his life.

Ideas about what should be in this book flowed from Bill; he was excited to partici-

11

pate and full of good stories. His answers to questions were succinct, yet rich in detail, as if he was in touch with that higher power that some writers allude to. Our chats struck just the right chords and triggered a flood of my own memories of our long friendship and, most importantly, of what I've learned from him.

Then again, much of the inspiration and driving force behind this book came from Bill Porter's fans. I've felt driven to introduce him to as many people as possible. I've seen and heard of many lives spiraling downward — physically, mentally, and spiritually — that suddenly improved when they read about Bill in the newspaper, saw him on a segment of ABC's *20/20*, or met him at one of our speaking engagements.

A common response to Bill's story is, "He made it through hardships I never dreamed of. What am I complaining about?" Admittedly, I had similar thoughts while juggling my role of mother to six children and writing this book, but visits with Bill always recharged me and kept me writing.

I met Bill when I was seventeen years old and still in high school. I walked into the school's administration office and my eyes were inexplicably attracted to a slip of paper tacked to the bulletin board. It read: *Delivery Person Wanted. Every other Saturday. Must supply own car. Please call Bill Porter at xxx-*

xxxx. I thought I already had a great summer job lined up, but something inside me said I must have this one. It sounded like a dream come true for a teenager, and it was! I cruised around in the family car, listened to the radio, delivered products, and made money. I even liked Bill Porter; he was a nice, hard-working man who paid me much better than the minimum wage.

Curious customers would ask, "What's wrong with Bill? Does he have MS or muscular dystrophy or what?"

At the time, I didn't know and I didn't know how to ask him. Besides, it really didn't matter to me because our relationship was friendly and profitable. Why risk one of the best summers of my life asking a question that might offend him?

Years later, after college and the birth of my first child, Bill's delivery person gave notice and he inquired about my whereabouts. I was flattered that he remembered me and wanted me back, and the extra money certainly would come in handy. Sure enough, our lives became inexplicably intertwined, and for more than twenty years we've watched each other fall down and get back up many times, all the better for the experience. Every time our lives hit a rut, Bill was there for me and I was there for him.

Often, if Bill wasn't physically with me during times of trouble, he was there in my thoughts, and somehow just thinking of him renewed me. I'd remember all he'd been through and how he turned negative situations into positive ones. Simply thinking of Bill lifted me, refreshed me, and allowed me to believe that I, too, could achieve my goals. I've talked to many fans of Bill who describe a similar phenomenon when they reflect on who he is and all he's accomplished despite his challenges. In this book, I hope to share the lessons I've learned from Bill Porter, so you may know him, too.

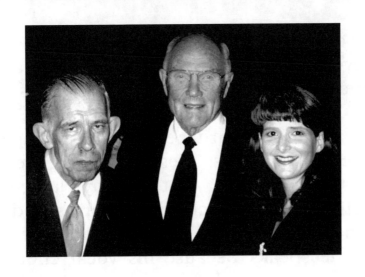

Chapter 1

Follow Your Passion

"Happy birthday to you! Happy birthday to you! Happy birthday, dear Bill! Happy birthday to you!"

I have never heard it sung so sincerely and by so many people. The entire audience at the John F. Kennedy Center in Washington, D.C. stood on their feet and applauded the sixty-sixth birthday of a most unsuspecting hero — Mr. Bill Porter, a door-to-door salesman for Watkins Products. Bill was all smiles as the clapping reverberated throughout the great hall. I, Shelly Brady, close friend and assistant to Bill, stood to his left; on his right stood another American hero, former astronaut and Senator John Glenn.

The occasion was the presentation of an achievement award from the National Council on Communicative Disorders (and Bill's birthday, of course).

Bill won the award because he managed to succeed in business despite having cerebral palsy, a condition that greatly affects his speech and the muscles in his arms and legs. Listeners must pay close attention to Bill when he speaks because his vocal chords release words in a halting pattern. Resist the temptation to finish sentences for him, however, because if one is patient the words do come and are well worth waiting for, especially if Bill is knocking on your front door with attaché case in hand. Bill was chosen for the award because he embodies the dreams, the spirit, and the hope of individuals with communication disabilities or diseases.

Was that the greatest moment in Bill Porter's life?

The convention center in downtown San Francisco echoed with the cheers of seven thousand men and women from fifty-six countries. They shouted one word in unison — a name, understood in all of the fourteen languages spoken here: "Bill, Bill, Bill, Bill." The stage lights were bright and Bill couldn't see their faces or their tears of joy, but he felt the emotion and the love of the audience, all members of the Million-Dollar Round-table. They represented the cream of the crop in the insurance and financial planning industries. When the cheers stopped, I spoke for about ten minutes on Bill's behalf because of his speech difficulties. The applause that followed lasted as long as the speech. Bill looked at me, as if asking for an idea as to when the standing ovation might end and what we should do in the meantime. I shrugged my shoulders and whispered, "Let's relish the moment."

Was that the greatest moment Bill Porter ever experienced?

The make-up girl applied powder to a shiny spot on the top of Bill's head. When ABC's *20/20* called about doing a segment on Bill, I nearly fell out of my chair. Here we were, a door-to-door salesman and his assistant, going about our rather mundane, day-to-day existence struggling to make ends meet, and all of a sudden ABC news correspondent Bob Brown is sitting across from us with the cameras rolling. Bill couldn't believe it when he found out that *20/20* had more than twenty million viewers. We were told the broadcast could change our lives. Companies would want him to share his story at their yearly conventions. I was wondering if there was a book or a movie in the future. Bill took it all in stride, only half-believing that the public exposure would help his sales; he knew that one-on-one sales work best. He was more interested in knowing, "Will I ever get to meet Barbara Walters?"

Was this the goal that Bill Porter had dreamed of?

The telephone rang. It was the personal assistant to the actor William H. Macy calling.

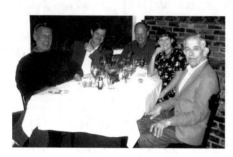

Macy and writer-director Steven Schachter wanted to fly to Portland to meet in person with Bill Porter and myself. After three long years of hard work and a handful of rejections, TNT was ready to produce a movie based on the life of Bill Porter. Bill Macy, an Academy Award–nominated actor, co-wrote the script and planned to portray Bill in the docudrama. I picked up Mr. Macy and Mr. Schachter at the Portland Airport, and since I'm a big fan of Macy's, I was trembling by the time they walked off the airplane. Soon, however, we were chatting like old friends. Then it was off to Bill Porter's house, where the two Bills met face to face. Macy extended his right hand to Bill, a gesture that was gladly accepted. To me, this handshake symbolized the great respect the two men held for each other. In an instant, I knew Macy was the right actor to portray Porter, and the sincere bonding between the two men brought tears to my eyes.

Was this the most exciting day in Bill Porter's life?

The palm trees swayed in the late afternoon breeze at the La Quinta Resort, a desert oasis outside Palm Springs, California. My pale skin was getting some color as we lounged by the pool, sipping virgin pina coladas.

"It doesn't get much better than this," Bill said to me as he adjusted his hat to keep the sun off his face.

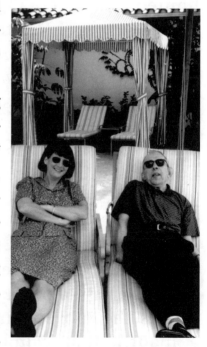

We were unwinding after giving a motivational speech to a few hundred conventioneers. It went well, and I figured Bill was finally getting used to life on the road. No more wet dreary winters in Portland, Oregon, slip-sliding his way up steep driveways and staircases. *So this is what it's like to be*

rich and famous, I was thinking; *I can handle this. I just need to figure the logistics of how I'm going to travel from resort to resort with six children and a husband in tow.* Bill brought me back to reality when he asked, "How many messages do you think are on my answering machine? I mean, how many orders? Some of those people are going to buy their products at a warehouse store if I don't get back soon."

"I doubt it," I said. "Those customers are loyal to you."

"Exactly," Bill replied. "Loyal to *me,* not an answering machine."

Today, for medical reasons, Bill's travel is limited and La Quinta is only a fond memory, but he often speaks of that trip to Southern California. He says he can close his eyes and feel the warm sun on his skin and hear the wind rustling through the palm leaves.

Was this what he had looked forward to doing all of his life?

Bill spent years pounding the pavement, knocking on doors, ignoring rejection after rejection. No matter what response he received after knocking, no answers or negative replies, he moved on, undaunted, for Bill had a mantra that calmed his nerves: "The next house will say 'yes.' The next house will say 'yes.' "

Bill repeated this chant over and over as he trudged up the hills of northwest Portland, approaching each house optimistically even if it was the same house that last month told him, "How many times do I have to tell you? Never, ever come back!" He'd go back again, month after month, with a fresh and confident attitude. It was all a part of his strategy, a strategy all good salespeople know about: wear them down until they tire of saying "no." Eventually, they will buy. Eventually, everyone buys.

Such positive thoughts constantly course through Bill's mind and body. *Did they just say something about not coming back? I must not have heard them correctly.*

After months and sometimes years of knocking on their doors, Bill finally breaks them down. First, he hears a hint of resignation in their voice. Next, they invite him in. Then, they agree to look at his catalog. And finally, it's "I'll take one of those." They may only order one bottle of vanilla this time, but it's a sale, a sale from someone who once told him, "No. Don't ever come back."

Was that the greatest moment? Yes, you bet it was.

When Bill is "cold calling" at a stranger's front door, he is in his element. This is the moment he lives for: not knowing who will answer, what their response will be, what mood they'll be in. But most importantly, he wonders this: Will I make a sale? Of his more than five hundred regular customers, Bill says that about thirty-five of them told him to never ever come back. They are among his best customers today.

Bill Porter has a passion for selling. His dream is to be number one. If there is one thing I have learned from him, it's that anyone can follow their passion and live their dream. Bill has proven to me that dreams have a way of coming true if we stay focused on the path, no matter what obstacles confront us.

Selling is Bill's life; he takes it with him wherever he goes. When companies first called wanting Bill to share his story with their employees, he had absolutely no interest. At first, I thought it was because he was embarrassed by his difficulty communicating. I later learned that he was uncomfortable not because of his speech impediment, but because speaking to a large audience wasn't his "style." He told me that he was a salesman from the old school, a one-on-one type of guy.

I, however, was very interested! Since I was a theater major in college, this was right up my alley.

"Wait a minute," I said. "Don't say no. We can do this speaking gig together."

Reluctantly, Bill agreed to give it a try for

my sake. What disturbed Bill more than stage fright was that the speaking engagements would cut into his door-to-door sales. Our first speech was scheduled for a Saturday.

"No way," Bill said. "Saturday is callback day." That's the day he telephones customers that weren't home during the previous week. I suggested that he double up and do callbacks the next weekend. After all, he was his own boss.

"Absolutely not," he said. "Period."

I tried another angle that I thought might work with him.

"Bill," I said, "suppose you make more money on Saturday from the speaking fee than if you stayed home and did callbacks?" He still wasn't swayed. Then it dawned on me.

"Bill," I asked, "what if we handed out catalogs to all three hundred audience members and invited them to be your customers? You could potentially double your sales next month." Bingo! I could see Bill calculating the sales figures in his head. And as it turned out, dozens of audience members purchased items from Bill after our talk.

Everywhere we go, Bill makes new friends and customers (these two words are synonymous to Bill). The first time we traveled abroad we were scheduled to fly to Calgary to speak to Bill's own company, Watkins, Inc.

The morning of our departure, a nagging thought kept crossing my mind. The night before, just before he dozed off, my husband asked, "Does Bill have picture ID?"

The question kept haunting me the next morning as I packed, said good-bye to the children, and caught a ride to the airport. Always prompt, Bill was waiting for me when I arrived. Together, we walked up to the ticket counter and presented our tickets. Then my nightmare came true. The agent asked, "May I see picture ID, please?"

"Here is my ID," I said. "However, my friend here has never driven a car. And, uh, well, therefore, he doesn't have picture ID."

Bill's fingers fumbled through his wallet searching for anything with a picture on it. Credit cards, bus passes, and various receipts soon littered the ticket counter. Finally, he held up his library card with the innocence of a child.

The agent was briefly amused, but quickly regained his composure and asked, "Does Mr. Porter have a passport or a birth certificate?"

"Yeah, but not with him," I said. "Say, do you subscribe to the *Oregonian*? You do? Great! Then you must know who this man is. He's the Bill Porter in the 'Life of a Salesman' article, the man born with cerebral palsy. The man who was told by the State of Oregon that he was unemployable, and who

24

went on to become the top salesman for Watkins Products. We have to get him to Canada to tell his story to conventioneers. Look at the picture of him on the cover of this magazine; underneath it says 'Bill Porter.' Doesn't that count as picture ID?"

The agent said he'd be right back; he had to speak to his supervisor. Bill and I stood nervously at the counter strumming our fingers and casting apologetic looks at the disgruntled travelers behind us.

Finally, the agent came back and said, "We can let you go to Canada, but you wouldn't be able to get back into the country without proof of citizenship." That could be a real problem for my husband and children, I thought. The ticket agent continued, "If you can secure proper documentation, we have a later flight."

We headed straight to a phone booth where I called the office of Vital Statistics in San Francisco, Bill's birthplace. After waiting on hold for ten minutes, I finally got a voice. "Yes, we can locate William Douglas Porter's birth certificate, but it will take three weeks to process. No, it can't be faxed. No, there's nothing we can do to satisfy the agents at the airport. Sorry." Click.

I chanted another of Bill's mantras, "I have no obstacles," as we hailed a cab and headed to Bill's house. We tore through drawers and closets. Old family photos distracted us from our mission of finding picture ID for Bill. "Look how beautiful your mother looks in this photograph. She was so pretty," I sighed. Quit gabbing and keep looking, I reminded myself.

At last, underneath a pile of scrapbooks, we found a worn paper bag with the word *Statistics* written in red letters. I dumped the contents on the floor and we sorted through them: death certificate for Ernest Porter, marriage certificate for Bill's parents, life insurance policy, old electric bills. Finally, something appeared with the words *William Douglas Porter* on it . . . a baptismal certificate. Maybe, just maybe, this would work.

I shoved everything into the bag and called a cab that took us to the Department of Motor Vehicles. After a twenty-minute wait in line, we stepped up to the counter. I placed the *Statistics* bag on the counter next to the magazine with Bill's picture on the cover. I pleaded our case.

"We missed our plane and we have to go to Canada. This is the famous Bill Porter and he needs picture ID."

I was just warming up when the DMV lady interrupted me.

"Oh, you're the man featured in the *Oregonian* article. I read that story and I couldn't stop crying." She paused a moment and looked at the documents on the counter in front of her. "What's this? You have only one piece of identification, your baptismal certificate. Hmm, you're really supposed to have two pieces of identification. If you promise not to tell a soul, I don't think there is any question who you are. Honey, you just come on back here and I'll take your picture. I'll have you on that plane in no time." Somehow, while I organized all the paperwork, Bill managed to sell his new friend/customer a can of Watkins cinnamon.

If Bill told you his version of this story, it would go something like this: *Once we missed a plane because I didn't have ID. Missing the plane didn't bother me at all; missing a day of selling is what annoyed me. Fortunately, all was not lost. The nice lady at the DMV bought a can of cinnamon and took a catalog to share with her family and friends. Boy, am I glad I didn't have picture ID; just think of all the new business I got. I wish Shelly would have calmed down; she looked like she was ready to pass out.*

Bill Porter is a perfect example of an individual succeeding because he stayed focused on something he felt passionate about. Like his father, Bill's passion was for selling, to be the best salesman he could be without compromising his values. Bill once received a ten-minute standing ovation at the end of one of our speeches when he passionately urged audience members to simply "go out there and make it happen." Following my passion was one of the first things I learned from Bill.

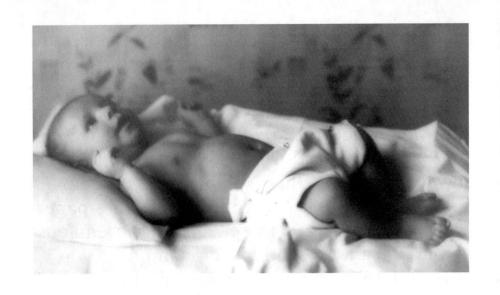

Chapter 2

It Doesn't Matter How You Got Here, Only Where You're Going

September 9, 1932, was the happiest day in the lives of Ernest and Irene Porter. The time was 2:20 A.M. and they were the proud parents of a baby boy, William Douglas Porter. In spite of the difficult labor (the doctor had to use forceps to extract baby Bill), Irene would have gladly repeated the experience for what they received that morning: a precious and healthy little boy. The birth certificate on the table was proof of that; on line 29, under the heading "Congenital Crippling Deformities," was typed the word "None."

I picture Irene with baby Bill in her arms during the first few months of his life, when no signs of cerebral palsy were evident. I see her counting ten fingers and ten toes, caressing his soft skin, and gently running her fingers over the handsome features of his face. He seemed perfect in every way.

It didn't take long, though, before she knew something was wrong. She knew it before anyone else. Bill's perfectly shaped left hand was always clenched ever so tightly. Irene also noticed that her infant son's back was arched and stiff. She spent hours massaging his shoulders and back. She gently pried his fingers open, only to see them revert back into a tight little fist.

On her own, Irene researched the stages of child development and discovered that Bill's growth was not proceeding normally. He wasn't strong enough to roll over, sit up, or crawl. He wasn't strong enough to hold the bottle on his own. Irene read every book she could find on child development, which, at the time, were few and far between. One book recommended what's called the "parachute test," whereby a baby is held level and face down, two feet over the bed, and dropped. By six months of age the baby should instinctively protect itself by spreading its arms and legs to ease the fall. Bill just plopped down on the bed without the slightest sign of self-protection.

Irene carefully watched the progress of infants of friends and relatives; she tried to objectively compare them to Bill's development. Shortly before Bill's first birthday, she couldn't deceive herself anymore; Bill was not performing as he should. She couldn't ignore the fact that Bill still clenched his left hand no matter how many times she tried to uncurl it. The hour-long massages weren't working the magic she hoped on Bill's poor posture. There was no denying that Irene and Ernest must seek a professional opinion.

Irene pointed out Bill's physical problems to the family doctor. The doctor immediately recognized the symptoms and diagnosed cerebral palsy. Suddenly, life was a whirlwind of doctors, therapists, and experts. Little was known about cerebral palsy in the 1930s, but most of the specialists suggested that Bill had no hope for a normal life. They predicted he would be mentally retarded and suggested he be placed in an institution. The Porters were appalled at the idea of their precious baby being torn from their lives. Irene knew in her heart that Bill was bright and intelligent. She vowed to do everything in her power to un-

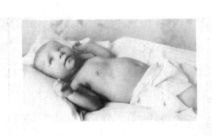

Greetings! FROM WILLIAM DOUGLAS PORTER.
Irene & Ernest

derstand and conquer the illness that crippled her son. Helping her son grow up to become the very best he could became her sole mission in life, *her passion.* No other children would be born in the Porter household; Ernest and Irene needed every bit of time and energy they could muster to ensure that Bill was well taken care of. They devoted their lives to Bill and never looked back.

Over the years, Bill asked his mother many times to repeat the story of his birth. She said, "It was a difficult labor that lasted far too long and everyone was afraid neither you nor I would make it. The doctor needed to use forceps because you were stuck in the birth canal. The very forceps that saved your life also damaged a section of your brain. That's why you have a difficult time using your muscles. None of that matters now; what matters is where you're going, not how you got here."

Bill had no idea of the pain Ernest and Irene felt upon the revelation that their son had cerebral palsy. Family members tell of the sadness they felt. Many tears were shed, and sometimes the questions "Why Bill?" and "Why us?" were asked. There never was a clear answer; they accepted it as part of God's plan. A close friend of the family recalls "The Porters were initially devastated when they learned that Bill had cerebral palsy, but it was only for a brief spell. Bill was their treasure, their gift from God."

Ernest quit his steady job as a salesman, a frightening prospect for anyone during the Great Depression, let alone someone with a child with a disability. He searched for work that would help him better understand and treat his son's disability. He found work with the Berry School in San Francisco, an educational institution for handicapped children. He worked in the physical therapy department and young Bill would often accompany his father to work. Bill fondly remembers trying on the "duck shoes," long boards roped to the feet of children who needed assistance in straightening their walk. Throughout the next decade, Ernest and Irene Porter worked at various locations of the Berry School — San Francisco, Los Angeles, Phoenix, and Chicago — wherever their services were needed.

Irene worked as a cook for the school. Her salary made up for the pay cut Ernest took when he left sales work. Ernest and Irene assisted Bill with exercises that greatly improved his muscle coordination. They also assisted Bill every evening with speech therapy. Bill learned quickly; his ability and will to communicate increased in leaps and bounds. Bill quickly proved naysayers wrong; his mental capabilities were normal. They were all on a long arduous journey, one that would determine whether Bill would stay with them or enter an institution.

No one except Bill really knew how he felt about his disability, if he felt inferior because he was different from the other children. Bill says he doesn't remember thinking negatively about his condition. He is blessed with inheriting a philosophy from his parents that believes in focusing on the future, not dwelling on the past. The past is something the Porter 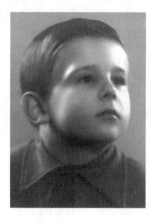 family learned from, not doted over. To Bill, his cerebral palsy is yesterday's news, something that isn't worth rehashing, and he doesn't want anyone else focusing on it either.

Several years after Bill and I first met, I finally got the courage to ask him about his condition. Although he set me straight about his cerebral palsy, his comments were short and to the point and the subject was not brought up again for another decade.

"I was just wondering," I asked awkwardly, "I mean, some of your customers, well, I wondered what you have. I mean is it MS or cerebral palsy or what?"

Bill matter-of-factly answered, "I have cerebral palsy."

I am rarely at a loss for words, but I continued to stumble forward. "What does that mean? How did you get it? Will it get worse?"

Bill replied, "I was born with cerebral palsy. My mother told me a doctor's instrument — forceps — damaged a section of my brain at birth. My condition will never get any worse, nor will it get any better. What you see is what you get. It's not a big deal. It's part of my past and it doesn't bother me. It doesn't stop me from accomplishing whatever I set my mind to . . . which happens, at this moment, to be doing well with the Watkins collection and doing even better in two weeks."

After doing some research on my own, I learned that cerebral palsy is frequently caused by a lack of oxygen to the brain, most often occurring during childbirth. Fortunately, accidents like the one that happened to Bill during childbirth are becoming rarer because of modern medical technology. Organizations such as United Cerebral Palsy have funded research into its causes and prevention. Pre- and post-natal care have greatly lowered the incidence of CP. I have often wondered if the forceps didn't damage his brain but instead saved his life since Bill might have been stuck in the birth canal, unable to breathe. Then I remember that it's senseless to ponder about Bill's CP; I must put it in the past, as Bill has.

As hard as I try, I just can't put myself in Bill's shoes. I can't comprehend how he maintains his optimism, how he enthusiastically gets out of bed on the coldest, dreariest mornings imaginable and prepares to hit the pavement. He has done this daily with vigor for more than thirty years. Every morning Bill's alarm rings at 4:45 A.M. so he has time to get ready to catch the 7:20 A.M. bus to downtown Portland. Bill needs this much time to look his best; he doesn't like to dress in a rush. He believes that appearance is essential in sales, especially in door-to-door sales where customers invite you into their homes.

And so the wee hours of Bill's mornings are filled with the painstaking process of dressing. His left hand doesn't help much with the putting on of socks, trousers, white shirt, blazer, and, finally, wing tip shoes. He always leaves the cuffs unbuttoned and his shoelaces loose. Occasionally, he has managed to accomplish these tasks alone, but usually they take too much time. Better, he has decided, to acknowledge his needs and ask friends at a downtown hotel for a little help.

In the past after Bill's best efforts, Irene would tighten his shoelaces, button his cuffs and collar, and clip his tie on. She would cook him a warm breakfast and pack him a lunch. That allowed more time for Bill to organize his paperwork and read the newspaper. For decades, Bill and Irene followed the same routine until she became ill with Alzheimer's. With much trepidation, Bill followed the doctor's advice and placed her in adult foster care and eventually in a nursing home. That's when Bill had to start relying on others to help him. Not being the most adept cook in the world, he learned to enjoy a breakfast of cold cereal and toast. He paid a neighbor to pack him a lunch.

Irene was a perfectionist when it came to housekeeping. When she was gone, Bill maintained her high standards: the bath towels were neatly folded and hung on the towel bar just so, the shrubbery was trimmed regularly, and the lawn edged, not just mowed.

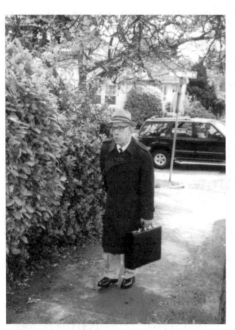

After getting help with his buttons, laces, and tie from the hotel bellhops, he was ready to catch the 8:30 bus to the West Hills, one of the better neighborhoods of Portland. Bill earned this prime territory by outselling other representatives of Watkins products.

It is now 9:00 A.M., more than four

hours since Bill arose, and he finally steps off the bus to begin his workday. Door after door he approaches, knocks or rings, and waits for an answer. He doesn't skip any houses on the presumption that no car in the driveway means nobody is home. Who knows? The car might be in the shop. Undaunted by no answer at most of the doors, Bill continues on, body slightly bent forward, left hand clutching a briefcase, right hand clenched in a fist behind him. His hat is squarely on his head, rain or shine. Often he wears a trench coat with a removable liner that is taken out in the spring and summer.

An eye checks out Bill through a peephole. He knows they are home, but they still don't answer. Other times, without even opening the door, he hears "No thank you." "I'm not interested." "I gave to charity last month." "We don't want any." "Go away." No after no after no, Bill treks on until at last someone is cordial and invites him in. Amazingly, the rejections don't bother him. They are all erased by a single order. Like a mantra, Bill repeats over and over to himself, "The next customer will say yes, the next customer will say yes." Eventually, Bill believes, they all will say "yes." He just has to be patient.

There have been a few very low points in Bill's life. A number of years ago, he was having a tough time making financial ends meet and became easy prey for a mortgage company soliciting his business over the phone. He signed up for an extremely expensive interest refinance package that nearly cost him his house. Because of the huge monthly payments, he had to cancel his medical insurance. Shortly thereafter, he had to have major back surgery. Between the medical bills and high house payments, Bill was almost forced into bankruptcy. It is only very recently, with the increased sales that occurred after the *20/20* show aired, that Bill has been able to pay off some of the loans and keep abreast of his medical expenses.

Bill made another financial blunder when he accepted an inflated estimate for work on his house. The company installed two basement windows and charged him $2,000. Fortunately, I happened to see the invoice on his table and questioned Bill about it.

"Did you get two or three estimates?" I asked.

"No, they seemed honest," was the reply.

I have come to believe an old saying: Sales people are the easiest people to sell to. I called the construction company and spoke to the owner, who acknowledged a billing error. He lowered the cost to a more reasonable $800. Now I try to scrutinize the bills on Bill's table before he pays them since he is incapable of adopting a suspicious attitude toward others. He always tells the truth to his clients: when they can expect delivery, what the total cost will be, and how the "satisfaction guaranteed" policy works. Since Bill never tells a lie, he assumes that others have the same regard for honesty that he does. When Bill and I were first trying to establish ourselves as inspirational speakers we were very naive. Early on we got an inquiry from a company on the East Coast. They didn't want us to go to the trouble of traveling — or so they said — and would gladly send a crackerjack team of journalists out to interview us in Portland. More than likely, they didn't want to go to the expense of flying us to their convention and putting us up in a hotel. I also knew the videotape wouldn't be as powerful as a live on-stage performance, but I didn't know how to convince them of the fact.

Well, before I knew it, the whole crew was at Bill's house. They interviewed and videotaped him without any monetary compensation. The video was then shown at their yearly convention to entertain and inspire the employees. I kept checking the mailbox, expecting some sort of compensation or at least a thank you note, but nothing arrived. To make matters worse, I misplaced the name of the company and wasn't able to let them know how I felt about what they had done.

For months, I was burned up that a company would take advantage of our innocence.

They knew speakers at business conventions are to be compensated, whether it is a live presentation or a videotaped one. I wasted a lot of time and energy fuming over this obvious wrongdoing. In fact, my anger and distrust were hampering the promotion of Bill and my new enterprise.

Bill took it all in stride; he was more interested in his next sale of Watkins Products. Finally, I followed his example and started believing that most companies are reputable and will pay fairly for our time and efforts. Eventually, we placed our trust in an agency that represents speakers. Now, little details such as getting paid for a speech are handled professionally. Who says Shelly can't learn a new attitude, can't learn from the past and yet leave it behind and live for the present and the future?

You see, I'm trying to apply Bill's way of living to my personal life. For a long time, I've carried a few bitter memories from my childhood. Raised by my mother and a physically abusive stepfather, I have sometimes bemoaned my less than ideal childhood. To this day, many of my brothers and sisters struggle with the effects of growing up in a dysfunctional family. With Bill as a role model, I am trying to accept the past and go forward. Occasionally, I lose my temper and can trace it directly back to painful experiences I had as a child, when my stepfather would burst into a fit of rage for no reason. Heaven forbid that I should subject my husband or children to ranting of that sort.

A lot of good things happened in my life, too. Eventually, my "wicked" stepfather changed: my family moved to Hawaii (that was rough!), joined a church, and adopted three children. Eventually, we moved back to Oregon where I met Bill Porter, then I met my husband and we created six amazing children. Life is beautiful.

If I could go back and change anything about my life, I wouldn't. I have come to realize that everything that's ever happened to me, both good and bad, has shaped me into who I am today.

Sometimes, I have days that are hard. I find myself reverting to past behavior patterns. I raise my voice impatiently or avoid helping someone. I make excuses to myself for my inappropriate actions: "I'm tired." "I had a rough day." "The house is a mess." Lately, I've been able to stop, turn myself around, and say, "It doesn't matter how I got to this point or where I am at this moment, only where I'm headed." I am learning to lower my voice and help children and friends in need.

Someone once said that it's better to be four feet from the mouth of hell headed toward heaven than to be four miles away from heaven headed toward hell. There are no fence sitters. You are either moving forward or backward. I think of my friend Bill, who in the past six decades has had his share of hard days. He knows his back will feel better, his migraine will go away, and he'll be able to catch his breath. It always happens. It always will.

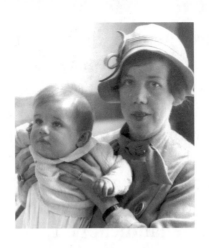

Chapter 3

Mother Knows Best

I shudder at the thought of how easily Bill's life could have turned out very differently, and how close we all came to not having the pleasure of knowing Bill Porter. The reason we know him boils down to one moment in time, more than half a century ago, a moment when a simple "yes" or "no" determined his fate. Instead of following the adamant advice of doctors, friends, and family and entering little Bill into an institution, his mother Irene made the decision to raise her son at home. She said, "Bill is my baby, my child. I will raise him," and stuck by her vow, for better or worse, in sickness and in health, for richer or poorer, rather than subject him to a life of lonely misery in a place where people don't get better.

Without taking anything away from Bill, the character traits that we most admire in him can be directly linked to his mother. It's difficult to imagine raising a child with cerebral palsy in the 1930s. Today there are high-tech wheelchairs, advanced prosthetic devices, and miracle drugs. Associations devoted to integrating the handicapped into mainstream society have helped make it illegal to discriminate against or inhibit physical access to individuals with disabilities. We are now more accustomed to seeing and interacting with mentally and physically challenged individuals than ever before.

Back when Bill was a child, no such technological or sociological advancements were 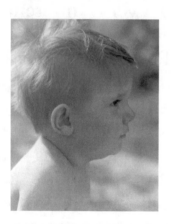 in place. It was extremely difficult for handicapped individuals to maneuver in stores and places of employment, let alone apartments and schools. At the same time, the social stigma attached to being handicapped could be devastating to an individual and their family. If a family decided to raise their "different" child at home, he or she was often hidden away from public view; poor education and rehabilitation often followed.

44

Irene Porter didn't buy into society's treatment of the handicapped; she rebelled against the prevailing attitude toward the disabled. She was a formidable foe to anyone who dared treat Bill as a lesser person because he had cerebral palsy. Her persistence and stubbornness is legendary among friends, family, and school administrators.

Bill, like other similarly challenged children, wasn't allowed in a public school until he graduated from an institution for the handicapped. Irene vociferously opposed this discriminatory rule; she saw absolutely no reason why Bill couldn't attend. Unfortunately, the school

Lincoln High School
Portland, Oregon
This certifies that
WILLIAM DOUGLAS PORTER
has completed the Required Course of Study as prescribed by the Board of Directors.
Given by School District Number One, Multnomah County, Oregon, on the 11th day of June, in the year of our Lord nineteen hundred and fifty-four.

district won the battle, and Bill was forced to graduate from the Grout School for Handicapped Children before he could attend Lincoln High School in Portland, where Irene promptly enrolled him when he reached the age of sixteen. Although Bill got a good education at Grout School, Irene felt it was important for him to receive a diploma from a public school if he was to get a decent job. Her determination and stubbornness paid off four years later when Bill graduated in a cap and gown at his high school graduation cere-

45

mony. He was a model student who paved the way for other handicapped students to enter public schools.

Irene knew that anything was possible if one is patient and persistent. She actually wrote the word "persistence" on slips of paper and secretly hid them in Bill's pockets or lunch bag for him to find later. Bill recalls a time in high school when he was trying his best to get an interview with the high school coach after the football team won a champion-ship game in overtime. Bill kept getting nudged aside by celebratory players and supporters. He was ready to give up and write the story without the one-on-one interview. On his re-porter's notebook he noticed the words "Per-

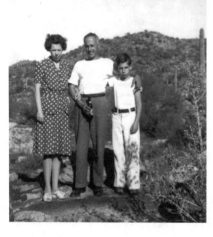

sistence pays off." Bill laughed aloud as he told me this story. Irene was up to her old tricks, but it kept Bill pressing on, which eventually got him a great interview with the coach that was featured in the next issue of the school paper.

Another character trait that Bill learned from his mother was neatness. Bill's cus-tomers are often surprised by how sharp he looks when making his route. Even though many of them are his friends now, Bill still dresses formally because he feels if he dressed more casually his sales might go down. I know where he got this passion for good grooming — Irene. Even on a tight budget she was a fastidious dresser; her blouses and skirts were always cleaned, pressed, and fashionable. Irene demanded the same of her son no matter how long it took him to dress. For years, Bill's fingers would trip over themselves as he practiced tying his shoelaces over and over again. His best efforts only got them tight enough to last a few minutes. Nevertheless, you can bet that before he approached his mother for help, he had done his best. Only then would she kneel down and tie them tighter. In fact, Irene was always willing to make the final buttoning of collars and cuffs, but otherwise her son was required to completely dress himself. Bill remembers the routine well:

"I had to wake up very early as a little boy, before my dad, even before the sun would rise. It took that much longer for me to get dressed. In the quiet stillness of the morning, I would struggle. My mom would busy herself with packing lunches and cooking breakfast. I learned to make my bed, pick up after myself, and get dressed just like every other child in the neighborhood."

Irene managed to keep herself and her

family well dressed because she was an excellent shopper. Once when I opened the clothes dryer at Bill's house, out tumbled six shirts with identical pinstripes. I asked him "Why don't you mix up your wardrobe a little and buy slightly different colored shirts? Maybe a beige one or a yellow one?"

"I didn't buy those, mom did," he answered. "They were on sale at the department store. Nice shirts, aren't they? Look, the buttons never fall off and the stitches hold together."

I didn't pursue the conversation further, except to agree they were of good quality. By using coupons and following sales, Irene managed to keep Bill and her family appearing to live well beyond their means. She was also an attractive woman, and when she dressed up she could turn quite a few heads.

Irene's attention to detail also was evident in the appearance of her home. Bill was assigned the task of keeping the yard neat, which was overwhelming at times for a child with physical limitations. I once asked Bill if he could ever remember his mom getting upset with him.

"Sure," he said, "she got upset a fair amount, like any mother does, right?"

Because I become cranky occasionally myself, I was glad to hear Bill's mom wasn't perfect. I can only hope when my children are grown, time will soften their memories and they'll be hard pressed to remember mom's occasional loss of patience. I won't hold my breath.

I prodded him further, "Do you remember any specific time?" One time in particular stood out in his mind.

"It was a warm summer day," he recalled. "My chore was to mow the lawn, weed the flowerbeds, edge the yard, and trim a few bushes. I started in the cool of the morning. After a lunch break, my mom inspected my progress and wasn't pleased. She thought I should have been nearly done, if not completely done before lunch. Instead, I'd hardly made a dent. This infuriated 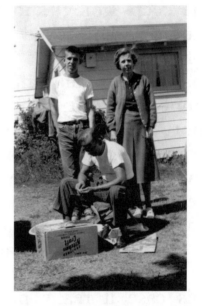 her so much she told me she was going to go take a nap, and that I'd better be done by the time she got up. Well, I wasn't done, and boy did she let me have it. She hollered and threw a real fit; she was so upset. She told me I was slow, too much of a perfectionist, and I'd have to stay right there in the yard and finish it even if it took all summer."

Bill insists to this day that he was working as fast as he could, but his mother hit the nail on the head when she accused him of being a perfectionist. Like mother, like son, you might say.

Bill always names his mother as his greatest inspiration. (His father played a much smaller role in Bill's life because he was gone much of the time, working as a salesman.) He thinks about his mother every day. On the days that are filled with pain or rejection, he keeps going, knowing she would be proud, knowing she loved him unconditionally. One of Irene's biggest worries was what would happen to Bill after she and Ernest were gone. She thus insisted that Bill learn to support himself and not depend on others. She wanted so much for him to be independent even though at times it contradicted her protective, motherly instincts. The Porters, like many families of that era, believed that hard work and determination could take you far. It was a lesson they passed on to Bill, and in his case it really paid off.

I can only imagine how Irene handled motherhood. When I became a mother, I was amazed by the little miracle in my arms, and at the same time overwhelmed. Nothing I learned in college prepared me for the awesome responsibility of parenthood. All I knew at that moment was I wanted to raise my children right and love them unconditionally, knowing someday I would have to let them go.

Six children later, I am still learning and

discovering the ups and downs, the disappointments, and, most of all, the joys of motherhood. My dream is to see my children mature, find their own paths, and become productive members of society. Some days, especially when they are squabbling and carrying on, I want this to happen sooner rather than later. Other days, I wonder where the time has gone. Who is this child, only moments before cradled in my arms, now fifteen years old with a driver's permit, backing out of the garage and forgetting to open the garage door? Most days, I try to enjoy the journey. Heck, it seems like yesterday when it was *my* mom who was tolerant when I backed the family car into a fence.

The greatest lesson I learned from Irene, which I think about daily, is the knowledge that unconditional love does exist. I learned how much power it has over both oneself and others. This purest form of love transcends nationalities, religions, and physical appearances. It isn't dependent on performance, grades, or physical prowess. I believe that Irene continuously enveloped Bill in tremendous doses of this kind of love, and it was this gigantic, all-knowing energy that enabled him to make it through the rough spots in his life. Bill carries this love around with him all the time. It has helped him to dismiss the prejudices and obstacles that would knock even the best of us down.

Recently, I experienced this type of love when I dropped my daughter off at high school. My older children are going through the stage when it's embarrassing to be seen with their mother. Half the kids drive themselves to school and anything less isn't considered cool. She begs me to drop her off two blocks away on a side street. On one morning, I rebelled. As she was getting ready to exit my car, I said, "Wait a minute. This is ridiculous. What are we hiding from?"

She replied with a long, drawn out, "Mom, you just don't get it."

I countered, "I do get it. I love you and

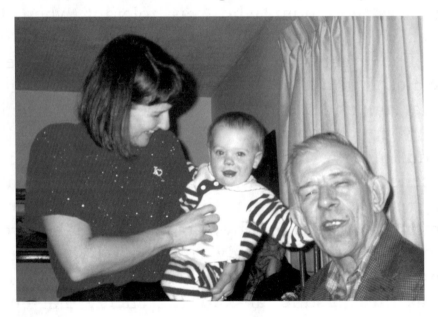

there is nothing wrong with that."

She stopped for a moment, rolled her eyes, and sighed. "I love you too, Mom. Next time, you can drop me right in front."

With that, she hopped out of the car and

walked toward the school. My heart swelled and tears came to my eyes as I remembered the feelings of love I experienced when she was first laid in my arms. It's important to me that my children know I will always be there for them and will always love them unconditionally. Thank you, Irene, for your beautiful example.

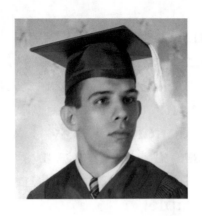

Chapter 4

Persistence Pays Off

Within days of Bill's extraordinary graduation from Lincoln High School in Portland, his father, Ernest, uttered three words that rang in Bill's head: "Get a job!" His father wasn't about to let Bill rest on his laurels. According to Ernest, the cap-and-gown affair was a significant achievement, but there was a real world out there, and he fully expected Bill to take an active and profitable role in it. To this day, when Bill repeats his father's strong words "Get a job," I sense the profound effect they had on his entire life. A little part of my motherly instinct disapproves of Bill's father acting so sternly and seemingly uncaring toward his disabled child, but another wiser part of me knows that Bill's father acted in the best possible way a parent can. I hope that I am as brave and unselfish when the time comes to set my children free to find their own paths.

Bill took his father's ultimatum to heart. However, his cerebral palsy shortened the list of employment possibilities. Gardening for neighbors seemed a logical choice; it didn't require the use of a car, and he always appreciated well-manicured yards. So Bill started knocking on doors and within one month he had a few yards under his care. He watered, mowed, and weeded, earning approximately four dollars a week, which seemed like a fair amount of money to Bill at the time.

Ernest thought yard work was below Bill, though, and rightfully so. Watering yards wasn't a real job, not for Bill; it wasn't fulfilling or challenging enough. Anybody could mow lawns. He agreed with his father. Besides, Bill wanted more human contact, not to mention higher wages. The fact was, he wasn't built for mowing, raking, and sweeping. Every work day ended in physical pain. His muscles contracted and his back stooped lower. He knew there had to be a better job out there, something that better satisfied his father and himself. Four dollars a week was fine if one lived at home for the rest of his life, but Bill had to consider that someday he would have to pay his own way and possibly care for his aging parents.

Bill's mother suggested that he consider being a salesman for United Cerebral Palsy. Irene had volunteered countless hours for the nonprofit organization throughout her lifetime. She hoped that one day a cure would be found. At the time, UCP was involved in a fund-raising drive in which people with cerebral palsy sold various household items and earned a small commission. Irene knew the fund-raiser worked and that it would be a great opportunity for Bill.

Bill jumped at the idea and soon was trekking throughout his neighborhood, knocking on doors, even approaching people on the streets and in parks. Customers must have liked Bill's enthusiasm for his products (and his life) because the nickels and dimes kept coming. He continued to water yards but avoided mowing them because he wanted to save his legs and back for sales work. After a few months, he was a top salesman for the local UCP affiliate. Finally, he felt like a contributing member of society. His father must have thought so, too, because he no longer told Bill to "Get a job."

After two profitable years of selling for UCP, Bill began to see a downturn in the market for his products; it was evident that customers could only use so many of the limited items he sold. In fact, Bill's best customers finally told him that they couldn't use even one more basket or potholder. Bill needed a product that was consumed or used up so he could get long-term repeat sales. He also realized that the hardest part of selling was developing a clientele who trusted and liked you.

"What a waste," he thought, "to develop all those good relationships with customers and not be able to sell them something they need on a regular basis."

Bill knew in his heart that he was a natural-born salesman; he simply needed the right product. Once again he brainstormed, searching for the perfect product to sell. As Bill explained to me, "The answer came to me as I noticed a mail order gift catalog my mother had been browsing through one day. Right in front of me was a booklet filled with products for sale. I flipped through the pages. There must have been at least a hundred different gifts. I wondered how I could sell these same items and make a profit. Then it hit me. It was so simple. I would cut out the pictures from the catalog, paste them on to construction paper, and then type in my own prices — higher, of course."

He didn't notice the hours and days slipping by as he cut, pasted, and typed each gift item, carefully creating a unique catalog for his sales venture. He wanted to make sure that if verbal communication broke down between himself and his clients due to his speech impediment, the illustrated catalog would do the explaining for him. Bill planned to visit his basket customers, his yard clients, and every home within a five-mile radius. He was hyped up to sell, sell, and sell again.

The venture paid off and Bill made more money than he ever had before. The fifties were a rosy decade for the Porter family. Ernest earned a comfortable living selling custom signs for the Ramsey Neon Sign Company. Bill had launched his own career as a salesman. Irene kept busy with household chores, the church, and volunteering for United Cerebral Palsy.

The sixties, however, were not so kind to the Porters. Ernest learned from his doctor that he had high cholesterol and should watch his diet. These early warnings from the doctor made Bill even more aware of his future responsibility as the main breadwinner in the family. The financial burden of caring for his father and mother began to weigh heavily upon his shoulders. He felt compelled to look for another job, possibly with a big name company, one that had health benefits and more opportunity for advancement.

Ernest never appeared sick and never missed a day of work, but Irene worried and fussed over him. He ignored the doctor's advice and continued to eat poorly. Bill knew it was only a matter of time before his family would have to make do on his meager income alone. But his gross pay of sixty-five dollars a month simply wouldn't keep food on the table. In the few free hours that Bill could spare each day, he searched for new and better employment. Thus began his daily trips to the Oregon State Department of Employment.

Every morning before his eight hours of selling would start, Bill took the bus downtown to meet with employment counselors. Day after day, week after week, month after month, he would walk the same blocks to stand in line behind dozens of other unemployed workers. Bill lists that experience as one of the most degrading and humiliating of his life.

Initially, the employment officers made a sincere effort to assist Bill. His attitude was excellent and his appearance was very presentable. When the position of stock clerk at a major pharmacy came up, they referred Bill. However, the cerebral palsy made his hands twitch in a most uncooperative way; he kept knocking the bottles and jars off the crowded shelves. Depressing as it was to be let go before his first day was out, Bill returned to the unemployment office the very next morning with his head held high and his shoes shined bright.

A few days later Bill's persistence paid off; another job offer appeared that seemed to be a perfect match. Goodwill Industries needed a cashier at one of their retail stores in downtown Portland. Bill was good with numbers and extremely honest. Unfortunately, his fingers wouldn't extend fully or respond accurately and he kept hitting the wrong keys. The manager of the store quickly lost patience with Bill's corrected register receipts, and he let Bill go three short days later.

Next, Bill was hired to work the docks at the Salvation Army, but it was soon obvious to everyone that Bill wasn't physically able to load the trucks. The well-meaning agents at the employment office finally realized that Bill couldn't be expected to perform well at jobs that required manual labor.

They told Bill they had found the right match and sent him to answer phones at the Veterans Rehabilitation Center. Bill couldn't figure out why anyone would hire him to do phone work considering his difficulties communicating, but he was willing to try anything they recommended. After all, they were the experts. After numerous complaints about Bill's slurred speech, he was let go from this job as well. With four job reports rubber-stamped with "Unemployable" in Bill Porter's file — the pharmacy, Goodwill Industries, Salvation Army, and the Veterans Rehabilitation Center — things were not looking up for Bill Porter's employability. His handicap was too limiting.

The agents at the state employment office

were cordial to Bill, but daily they came back with the same depressing news: "Sorry Bill, nothing today." Bill persevered day after day, week after week, and month after month. There simply was no work in which Bill's handicap wouldn't impair his performance. Finally, after five grueling months, an agent politely told him that he didn't need to come back. The state deemed him unemployable; they recommended he stay home and collect disability. The agent went on to tell Bill, "You have too much motivation for your own good." To say the least, Bill Porter did not take this as a compliment. He took it as a direct challenge to his self-worth, a personal challenge, as did his parents. He vowed to prove them wrong.

Bill stopped going to the employment office and decided to be his own employment counselor. That meant screening the Help Wanted ads of the Portland *Oregonian* on a daily basis. Everyday he would call a half dozen job possibilities. But most of the people he spoke to wouldn't let him complete the phone interview, let alone come in for a personal interview. Sometimes the company representative would harshly state that they weren't hiring as soon as they heard his speech impediment. He would often hear the abrupt click of a phone being hung up on him, but the dial tone only prompted Bill to call another ad.

Undaunted, Bill pressed on, ignoring any jobs that required manual labor. And then, like father, like son, he decided to focus on sales jobs. He knew he could sell; the experience with UCP had taught him that. One of the first companies he contacted was the Fuller Brush Company. He was amazed and his spirits soared when the local distributor said he would stop by for a personal interview. Bill relates the story this way:

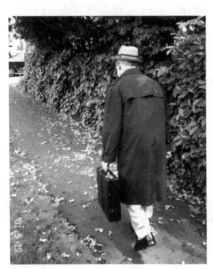

"The Fuller Brush man came into my living room and before we even had a chance to talk much, he said the job wasn't for me. He had a black case with him — the product bag — but told me I wouldn't be able to carry it. He didn't even ask me to try. He just took one look at me and assumed I couldn't do it. I knew he didn't want me. He wouldn't even give me a chance."

Bill and I have repeated this story at speaking engagements across the country. I always look at him when we're done — he gets a twinkle in his eye whenever he hears the story — and ask, "Have you ever noticed the Fuller Brush Company hasn't invited us to speak?" He quickly answers with a big grin and giggles. Bill's giggles are so sincere and so contagious that soon the entire auditorium is filled with laughter.

However, if a Fuller Brush representative, or a representative from any of the other companies that turned down Bill's services, is reading this, please don't be concerned. We realize that these incidents were a long time ago and that employment practices have changed considerably since Bill was turned away. We now know that most of those companies that rejected Bill wish he were on their team. And yes, we would welcome an invitation to share Bill's story with any and all of them, the Fuller Brush Company included!

So Bill ignored the rejections and called the next ad for a sales position — Watkins, Incorporated. They, too, agreed to interview Bill in person. This time Bill wasn't about to take "no" for an answer. He met the Watkins director's reluctance to hire him head on.

"I know I can do this job," he told him. "I've been successfully selling for the past ten years. It's in my blood. My father is a successful salesman. It almost doesn't matter what product I sell, customers enjoy buying from me."

Once again Bill waited for the rejection. It was only a matter of how it would come. Would it be the familiar "Don't call us, we'll call you" or "The position has already been filled"? The manager took his time. Finally, with great hesitation, he offered Bill the job, on a trial basis only. So what if it was the worst territory in Portland. It was a real job! It was a lot better than disability payments, and it was certainly better than mowing lawns.

Within a week of the job interview Bill had equipped himself with a briefcase filled with colorful catalogs and optimistically hit the streets of his new territory. His elation quickly turned to dismay, however, as he walked from house to house. The neighborhood was worse than he had imagined: caved-in porches, missing steps, handrails hanging by a nail. Most of the houses desperately needed paint and the yards were unkempt and overgrown. No wonder the manager gave him a crack! Since the job paid commissions only, the company had nothing to lose. Bill doubted if anyone had *ever* made a sale in this neighborhood. It was a wonder the United States Postal Service even delivered mail here. Forget that he wasn't going to make a dime; he might get hurt falling through a porch! Stubbornly unwilling to survive on disability payments, he climbed step after rickety porch step.

Rejection after rejection only made Bill more determined to prove he was employable, that he was a salesman. He would make his parents proud. Watkins wouldn't regret hiring Bill Porter. Still, he couldn't believe there were so many excuses for not buying a good product from a good salesman. "We're moving." "We don't have any money." "No soliciting." To Bill, every "no" simply meant that the first "yes" couldn't be many doors away.

At the end of his first day, he returned home, having sold nothing. Refusing to give up, he sat down to learn more about the products he was selling. Perhaps if I learned more about these Watkins products, he told himself, I could really believe in them and share that belief with others. Then they would buy them!

Hour after hour passed as he tried to memorize every item and price in the catalogs. What size boxes does the laundry detergent come in? Is the cinnamon really the freshest on the market? Is it cheaper and wiser to sell the large size? What's my commission? Based on the literature, Bill decided he could be proud of what he was selling. But it wasn't until Bill came to the sentence "Watkins, Inc., backs their products with a 100 percent money-back guarantee" that his enthusiasm really soared. The implications to Bill were huge. What a sales tactic! He pictured himself promising an unsure customer that if they weren't 100 percent satisfied with their order, they could get their money back.

In other words, the customer wasn't risking anything.

He called the district manager the next day to verify that the company really would refund a customer's money if they weren't satisfied. The manager answered "Yes," unaware that Bill intended to use this guarantee to the fullest extent possible. If Watkins, Inc., was so sure customers would love their vanilla extract that they had the guarantee etched right onto the glass container, then surely this was a great product that was almost never returned. Theoretically, a customer could even use up to one-fourth of the bottle and still get a refund! If Watkins was that confident about their products, then Bill certainly should be. He decided to project that confidence and enthusiasm as part of his sales presentation. He could hardly wait to hit the streets. He knew he would make a sale.

Bill tells the story of his first sale as if it happened yesterday, when in fact it was more than four decades ago.

"I wasn't doing too well selling in that first territory until I came upon an apartment building. I had a good feeling about the place. Unfortunately, I couldn't get into the building. Every entrance was locked. I didn't know what to do, but I knew I had to get inside. Then I got an idea. I decided to hide just inside the porch behind a pillar. When someone came along to open the door, I would grab it before it shut and sneak in."

And Bill did exactly that. He started knocking on doors inside that building and finally made his first sale on the third floor. In complete honesty, he assured the lady that she would get her money back in full if she wasn't satisfied with the way the cleanser worked. "Okay," the lady said, "where do I sign?" Eventually Bill made quite a few new friends and customers in that building. Persistence finally paid off for Bill Porter. His mother would be ecstatic.

Unfortunately, Ernest Porter passed away in his sleep on September 8, 1962, one day before Bill's thirtieth birthday and only five months after Bill won his first sales award. Father and son never took the time to talk about his success. Bill doesn't remember why their lives had drifted apart. Perhaps

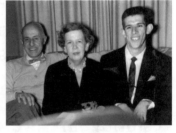

they were both too busy working. Bill would always struggle with his feelings about his father, always wondering if his job with Watkins satisfied the man who etched into Bill's brain the command "Get a job." Would Bill still hear those words if his father was alive today? Regardless, what mattered most then was that he now had a job and he was going to keep it. He also was going to excel at it beyond his father's wildest dreams. Bill was the man of the house now, and the sole provider for his mother.

It was sheer determination that landed Bill his job at Watkins, Inc. Eventually, he became the top-selling Watkins salesman in the entire Northwest, a position he continues to hold today.

Bill's amazing persistence is one of many character traits that admiring fans often mention in their numerous cards, letters, and e-mails. Readers report that they are better able to persevere through their own day-to-day and lifelong problems after they hear Bill's stories. The Brady family is no exception. Our fourteen-year-old daughter, Katrina, was diagnosed with PVNS (pigmented villanodular synovitis) in 1998. In layperson terms, this rare disease is essentially a reoccurring benign tumor within the knee joint, resulting in severe pain and limited mobility. Thankfully, PVNS is not life or limb threatening; the doctors have operated on her five times since the diagnosis to remove the tumor. We hope the last procedure will finally stop the growth, but many more surgeries may be in her future.

As you can imagine, Katrina's disease and physical handicap is at times devastating and incomprehensible to her. On the way home from the last operation, with her leg in a brace and crutches in the back seat, I glanced over to gauge her mental state, figuring that she would be completely depressed and in need of encouraging motherly words. To my surprise, she was looking out the window with a smile on her face. I remarked, "I'm glad to see you're handling this so well, honey." She replied, "I was just thinking of Bill."

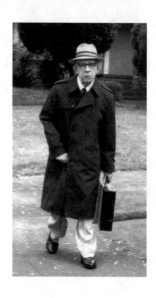

Chapter 5

Don't Take "No" for an Answer

According to the *Merriam-Webster Dictionary*, the word "no" is an act or instance of refusing or denying something. For instance, a customer's refusal to purchase goods or services from a salesperson is generally expressed via the word "no." For some reason or another, Bill Porter doesn't hear it that way. Bill hears the word "no" differently; he hears it to mean that the customer will be glad for Bill to return at a more convenient time or pleased to be shown another, more necessary product.

"No" is a powerful word used by children, parents, educators, and business associates.

How one relates to it is shaped in early childhood, where many of us learned only the literal dictionary definition of the word. In adulthood, many of us still fear the word, and sometimes unhealthy or unstable relationships can be damaged or destroyed when a "no" is heard from someone close to us.

I learned from Bill Porter that when someone says "no" they are simply asking you to modify your proposal or change your delivery. I believe that Bill's attitude toward the word "no" and his ability not to focus on the "negative" are traits that many people admire in him.

Some have interpreted Bill's cerebral palsy as one gigantic "no" dished out by the heavens, but he never looked at it that way. I have to admit there was a time when a blemish on my face before a Saturday night dance felt like more of a handicap than Bill's cerebral palsy was to him his entire life. When he could have collected disability or at least taken a job that wasn't so mentally and physically demanding, Bill chose instead a profession — door-to-door sales — that challenged his so-called "handicap."

Bill's association with Watkins began in December 1961. Expecting the worst, the district manager gave Bill a territory in Portland that no one else wanted and where sales were almost nonexistent. The houses were run-down and many households were so strapped for cash that anything Bill had to offer for sale was considered a luxury.

"It was hard to sell there because many of the people weren't home," Bill recalls. "They were all working to make ends meet. There were times I felt like quitting but knew I couldn't."

Bill managed to eke a meager income out of this poverty-stricken area. However, he and his mother worried about Ernest's health and the possibility of a day when his father would no longer contribute to the family income. Bill knew it was time to pursue a more lucrative territory or get another job. He approached his district manager with an idea.

"What if I took the territory near my home, the one where I sold baskets for United Cerebral Palsy? What if I sold Watkins products there? I already have a client base." The manager told him the territory belonged to someone else. Bill was ready for that one.

"According to the research I've done, Watkins doesn't have a policy concerning territories." Bill was right. At the time, territories were loosely defined and assigned; salesmanship and performance weren't determining factors. Bill thought his track record should be taken into account, as well as his proximity and knowledge of the area. The manager's answer was a flat-out "No. The territory is taken."

This didn't quell Bill's need and desire for a better territory. He figured he simply had to present more compelling logic to the manager. A week later Bill approached him again.

"It wouldn't really be like I was stealing someone else's area. It would be more like I was getting my old territory back, like a re-union. You know it's the territory where I belong."

The manager said he needed a few weeks to think about it. Bill knew he had a foot in the door. Next time, he would close the deal.

At their next meeting, Bill flatly stated, "I'll sell more Watkins products than anyone in the history of Portland. I know I can do it. Just think of the money Watkins will make — and you, too — since you make commissions on what I do."

Reluctantly, the manager gave in to Bill's request. Bill told him he would never regret it. In fact, it only took three months in his new territory for Bill to become a member of the Watkins $1000 Club, an achievement for which he received an impressive certificate. Irene framed it herself and proudly displayed it on the wall. Two months later, Bill was featured in Watkins News. The following article appeared in the July 9, 1962 issue:

PORTER POSTS $1076 SALES MONTH, KEEPS PACE WITH TOP PORTLAND DEALERS

Bill Porter of North Portland, Oregon, showed during May that with the help of sales aids, a determined effort, and spending eight solid hours, five to six days per week, in face-to-face selling, profits come comparatively easy. A good indication of this was his $1076 total for the month and an impressive $340 for the short Memorial Day holiday week.

Since becoming a dealer in December 1961, he has consistently followed Company-suggested sales methods and has placed primary emphasis on the liberal use of Catalogs and Free Gifts. During the month of May he purchased five full cases of Catalogs and had a young boy strew them in his locality.

Due to a handicap, Porter is unable to drive a car and he therefore walks upwards of seventy blocks from his home to his locality in a six-day week. According to Distributors Ted and Isaac Marto, Porter's eight-hour day begins when he reaches his locality, not when he leaves home. Porter has achieved his remarkable sales despite a physical handicap and a speech impediment. Division Manager C. C. Hunter says about Porter: "It's amazing that Porter can come forth with such outstanding sales. It's no small wonder that he puts other dealers to shame."

Irene Porter was immensely proud of Bill's achievements. She clipped the newsletter article and carried it in her purse. Bill still blushes when he tells the story of Irene bragging to friends and neighbors about the article, as if he'd been elected the president of Watkins.

Ernest and Bill never did discuss Bill's achievements, and to this day I sense that Bill still feels a little cheated; he wishes his dad had at least shook his hand or given him a pat on the back.

The accolades Bill received from corporate headquarters inspired him to work harder. The certificate and the news article were proof positive that Bill was a great salesman. He awoke every morning confident that he would sell more than the day before, and he carried this positive attitude throughout each day. The following statement from Bill is a good example of how he focuses on the positive, rather than the negative.

"If there were ten houses on a block, I would go to each one of them. It didn't matter if some families took better care of their yards or cars than others did. In each one lived a potential customer. If people in eight of the ten houses told me no, I wasn't discouraged because that meant two families bought from me. In three months when I covered that block again, I would go to all ten houses. Some salespeople would only go back to the houses they had successfully sold to. Not me. I knew that eventually people in each of those eight houses would buy from me, and many did! I knocked on the front door of every house in my territory about once every three months. Eventually, I built up to more than five hundred regular customers."

Every day, Bill would knock on doors for

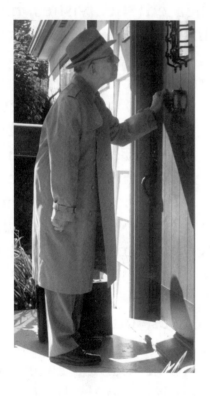

eight hours, covering seven to ten miles on foot, rain or shine. He knocked at approximately one hundred homes per day, and if he was lucky, one in ten would buy something. Other days he might have as few as five orders at the end of his beat. If he was fortunate enough to get beyond the usual "Not interested," he knew he was on his way to a sale. If someone invited him in, it was a done deal for sure.

Mrs. Brown is now a regular client of Bill's, but for years she resisted. There was a time she told Bill to never come back because there wasn't a chance in heaven that she would order anything in his catalog. Mrs. Brown was flabbergasted when he would show up every three months just to make sure she wasn't running short of something like cinnamon or laundry soap. One day Mrs. Brown reluctantly let Bill into her house. His timing happened to be perfect because he discovered that she was running low on vanilla and it was just before Thanksgiving. She remembers, "Bill had it all figured out. He wouldn't leave until I bought something. He'd just keep showing me products until I saw something I really needed."

Bill has a special fondness for Mrs. Brown. "Out of my five hundred steady customers," he says, "about forty are people who told me they didn't want anything and to never come back. Today, they are some of my best customers! Mrs. Brown was one of those forty."

Bill has the memory of an elephant when it comes to remembering when his customers are out of essentials. He knows, for example, when Mrs. Brown's bottle of window cleaner is starting to suck air. One customer relates that when Bill visited her in May he was set to write her up for a box of detergent. She politely explained that the family would be gone for three months on vacation, camping, and visiting relatives. They would use laundromats and wouldn't need detergent until they got back. She asked Bill when he would be back in her neighborhood and expected a very approximate answer such as "sometime in the fall."

"I'll be back the morning of August nineteenth," Bill replied. Exactly three months later to the day, Bill appeared on her doorstep, order book in hand, ready to write up the detergent. She can't say she was too surprised, since Bill managed to sell her some insect repellent before she left on vacation!

Over the many years I delivered products for Bill, I came across a few customers who would pull me aside and ask for help. They had placed orders with Bill on the spur of the moment because they liked his enthusiasm and upbeat attitude, but they later realized that they didn't need them. They just didn't know how to say "no" to Bill, and when they did he didn't seem to hear them; he just kept showing them new Watkins products. Their cupboards were filled with jars and boxes of unopened spices, pasta, and bagel mixes. Bill could sell soup mixes to people who ate every meal out and meat tenderizers to vegetarians. I'd just shrug my shoulders, wish them luck, and say, "See you next time."

After many years of watching and learning from the pro, I am finally able to proclaim that I have learned to adopt and institute Bill's attitude towards negativity. Numerous times, at critical junctures in my life, I have said to myself, "If Bill Porter refuses to take 'no' for an answer, why should Shelly Brady?" And like magic, it worked! Since I started adopting this new attitude, my personal and professional life has blossomed. Doors to opportunity that were always shut have suddenly swung open. The following story illustrates just such a door opening.

Bill and I have spent the last few years traveling and sharing his story with companies all over the world. Audience response has been terrific, and requests for our services have been phenomenal. However, our enterprise hit some rocky roads during its start-up. When businesses first started calling to book us, Bill said, "No! No way!" As far as he was concerned, he was a salesman, not a public speaker. So in the finest Bill Porter style, I replied, "Wait a minute, Bill. This is right up my alley. You're forgetting that I majored in theatre. I love the stage. Besides, the publicity might help 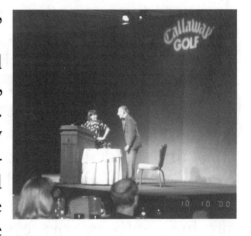 sales." Bill suddenly grew quiet; he may very well have been crunching numbers. A few moments later Bill agreed to participate in at least one speaking engagement. Many more followed, of course.

Our enterprise has been a dream come true for me: following my passion, speaking and inspiring others. I am constantly amazed by how many hearts are touched by Bill's story. Being a bit of a showman himself, Bill loves the attention but is more impressed with how his sales of Watkins products have skyrocketed since becoming a celebrity.

The year 2000 was unbelievably busy for Bill and me. The previous year had been filled with presentations, writing the first draft of this book, interviews, and a television movie deal. Bill continued to service his door-to-door Watkins accounts even though he could now afford to live off his speaking income. I somehow managed to keep my family life in order despite flying off to speaking appointments and meeting with movie producers, all the while toting child number six in my belly. When an agency specializing in booking speakers approached with a desire to represent us, I was ecstatic. Up to this time, I'd been managing all aspects of our tours: the airline flights, the hotel reservations, and the presentation itself. However, signing with a professional agency has its pluses and minuses. Spontaneity and improvisation had to be kept to a minimum. When the agency booked, we had to be willing, ready, and able. We polished our presentation and included video clips. Bill and Shelly were going Hollywood!

Our agent scheduled a presentation with Williams Communications in January of 2000. Since I would be eight-and-a-half months pregnant at the time, my husband, John, agreed to accompany Bill on the trip. I videotaped my portion of the presentation and our agent was satisfied that all would go well. However, just days before Bill and my husband were to fly to Orlando, Florida, Bill complained of not feeling well and that he was having breathing difficulties. I thought his complaints were psychosomatic because I wouldn't be by his side.

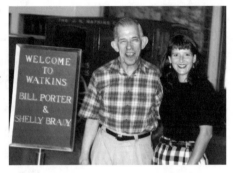

Our relationship with the speaking bureau appeared to be ending before it began. What's a mother to do? The five previous pregnancies were never more than three days early, so the odds were that I would be home well before labor began. And so against the doctor's orders and airline policy, I decided to join Bill and make the trip to Orlando. But this didn't pacify him; now he was worried about my health as well.

Two days before we were scheduled to fly out, Bill decided he simply wasn't feeling good enough to make the trip. I felt in my heart that Bill was physically okay. Yes, he

81

suffered from acid reflux due to pain medications he'd taken after an accident three years before. The doctors did manage to get the acid reflux under control, but due to his cerebral palsy some of the acid had dripped into his lungs, scarring them, and he had to use an inhaler twice a day. Other than an occasional episode when he couldn't catch his breath for a few moments, he got along fine, running his errands, selling, and traveling. I begged and pleaded with Bill to try and make the trip. He simply refused.

My world seemed to come to an end that night. I couldn't sleep, one minute sobbing into my pillow about my outcast state, the next minute stoically facing the reality that my life as a speaker was over. On the one hand I was sad because Bill's inspiring story wouldn't reach an audience that wanted to hear it, and on the other I was selfishly depressed because my own dreams were going down the drain. I loved the stage, the lights, the cameras, and the applause.

The next morning I decided out of desperation to try the Bill Porter don't-take-no-for-an-answer approach to a problem. I phoned our representative at the agency to sell them on a novel approach to the dilemma. What if I flew to Orlando without Bill and, using the latest audio-video technologies, he appeared on screen via satellite feed, much like at the Academy Award Ceremonies when the winner is unable to attend? It all made perfect sense to me because when we signed with the agency we talked about the future and how the day would come when Bill would no longer be up to traveling and speaking. Things would simply get speeded up, that's all! However, our agent had hoped to establish Bill and I as speakers together for at least a year or two before I appeared alone. He certainly didn't anticipate Bill's inability to fulfill his commitment with one of the agency's best clients.

I persisted and explained to our agent that we had little to lose at this point. If I went "belly-up" (pun intended) on stage and the clients wanted their money back, so be it. We'd survive. Bill still had Watkins products to sell and I had my family. The conversation ended with an "I'll get back to you."

Within an hour our agent phoned and asked how soon I could pack my bags — I was on my way to Disney World (and hoping that child number six would wait until I got back). The presentation went well with me alone on stage and Bill live in the background on large screen television via satellite. Williams Communications was so pleased they invited us to speak again two months later in Las Vegas (this time with baby in tow). This invitation came with full knowledge that Bill might not be able to make it in person. As it turns out, Bill's health took a turn for the better, and we continued with our scheduled speaking engagements for the next few months. One of the conference planners was so touched by Bill's story that she approached him with the idea of being the spokesperson for Williams Communications. Bill was flattered, but the timing was wrong and the deal never panned out. He found it ironic, though, that he was once fired for not communicating well over the telephone, and now here he was being considered for the position of spokesman for a major communications company.

Bill knew his traveling days would be over sooner than I wanted them to be. As romantic as life on the road sounds, it takes a toll on the body and the spirit. Dorothy of *The Wizard of Oz* was right when she said, "There's no place like home." Airports, ground transportation, hotels, and restaurants all take their toll. They are especially tough on a person as well organized as Bill; his success is based on a well-orchestrated daily routine.

On another much-anticipated trip, Bill reluctantly told me he couldn't come along, and I knew he was really suffering. Bill's doctors even recommended that he take some time at home to regain his full health.

The situation was very distressing to our client. Many of the conventioneers had bought tickets in anticipation of meeting the main feature, Mr. Bill Porter. The agency's reputation was also on the line; contractually, they had agreed that Bill would appear in person at the convention. Bill's name was in bold-faced type on the program. Attendees were flying from all over the country to see and hear Bill Porter, not Shelly Brady.

When our agent called the person in charge to break the bad news about Bill's health, offering me as a consolation prize, the door slammed shut. The promoters of this convention were not as flexible as Williams Communications. The answer was a re-sounding "No Shelly without Bill." My life as a speaker once again appeared to be over.

In another one of those Bill Porter moments, I got an idea. I called the convention organizers directly and told them I was confident I could share Bill's story myself with Bill possibly linked via satellite or telephone. I assured them I did it previously and it was very well received. I told them I would personally lay my speaking fee on the table. They could pay me whatever they felt my presentation was worth, even if it meant I'd get nothing. I was confident they had to accept my offer. I felt like Bill Porter telling a Watkins customer, "Satisfaction guaranteed or your money back." On top of that, I wasn't about to take "no" for an answer.

The chief organizer of the convention agreed to consider my offer and promised to get back to me. My agent was on pins and needles, and probably searching for new clients. An hour later the phone rang. Yes, the company would take me up on my offer. I would attend and speak in person with Bill connected via telephone. They would determine our speaking fee once it was over and the audience response was evaluated. I called my husband at work to tell him I was leaving town the next day.

"I'm not surprised," he remarked. "Nobody says no to you, dear."

Or Bill Porter, I thought. Two weeks later, a check arrived for the full speaking fee.

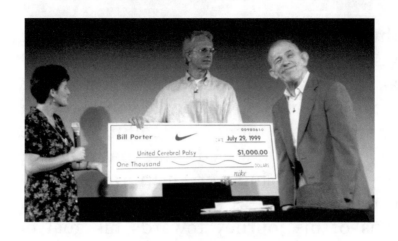

Chapter 6

Know Your Limits and Reach Beyond Them

At the 1996 Watkins International Convention in New Orleans, Bill Porter received a standing ovation when he closed the meeting by telling the audience, "Go out there and do the best job you can." The theme of the convention was "Achieving Goals," and the meetings and speeches promoted the belief that seemingly impossible goals can be realized by assessing one's limitations and reaching beyond them. Bill is living proof of that ideal.

Some of us are lucky enough to know exactly what our goals are, which, according to Bill, means the battle is half won. He believes great experiences and memories line the pathway leading towards the achievement of goals. Once you know in your heart your goal is the right one, even small steps toward achieving it will give you a sense of accomplishment. Bill found his calling — sales — early on and followed that path no matter how steep the hills or deep the valleys. He can recount endless stories about the ups and downs of his journey towards his goal of becoming a first class salesman.

Bill's attitude about setting and achieving goals can be traced to his youth when he developed a passion for sports. He smiles broadly when he talks about listening to baseball games with his parents, when they would all sit around the dining table next to a huge radio. That was before the days of television, when active imaginations were necessary to visualize all the action.

Bill still cherishes his scrapbook of autographed pictures of the New York Yankees. (He wrote the team manager asking for an autographed baseball and received photos instead.) Bill and his folks followed all professional sports, and visitors to the Porter household knew a lively discussion about the pros and cons of various teams and the players was inevitable. Many nights before Bill went to sleep, he imagined himself playing sports. He dreamed of hitting a grand slam or throwing the winning touchdown. Sadly, the fact that he had cerebral palsy always snapped him back to the reality that his physical limitations prevented him from even joining the neighborhood boys at the local sandlot.

When Bill entered high school, he found a way to circumvent his condition and enjoy sports as much as other children. He asked the coach if he could be the team's water boy, and the coach gladly obliged because nobody else wanted the task. At every game, Bill passed out towels and filled water cups for the active players, but he didn't stop there; he got the idea of making himself the official keeper of team statistics. "The day before the game," he remembers, "I'd type all the players' names in a column and the different plays across the top. I'd bring my paper and pencil to the game and mark each play by the appropriate player. Each night after the game, I would stay up half the night typing up the stats to give to the coach the next day."

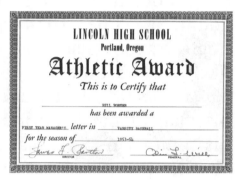

Later, Bill worked as a sports writer for the Lincoln High newspaper. In his column, he wrote about the highlights of the game, followed by the complete statistics. His column was titled "Porter's Tips." His contributions to sports at Lincoln High School were much appreciated, and he was awarded with a letter jacket at the senior banquet. Today, the jacket is one of his most prized possessions and it still hangs in his closet, ready to be modeled by Bill for anyone who asks about it. The 1954 yearbook for Lincoln High School lists Bill Porter as the "most likely to become a sportswriter for the *New York Times*." Bill successfully accomplished his goal of participating in sports by knowing his limitations and reaching beyond them. He cherishes his sports memories at Lincoln High School as much as any varsity quarterback.

In the 1980s, Bill and I both learned a sobering lesson about the limited time one has here on this earth when his mother, Irene, exhibited early signs of Alzheimer's disease. Bill remembers the moment clearly:

"It started out of the blue. One day I was getting ready to go to work and my mother started complaining. She hadn't been feeling well and she said I was a terrible son for going off and leaving her alone. I didn't know what to do. I knew I had to go to work. I had to pay the bills. She would be fine for a few days and then it would start all over again. Mother would cry when I left in the mornings and when I got home she wouldn't speak to me for a couple of hours."

It was the most excruciatingly painful experience in Bill's life. His heroine and biggest supporter seemed to be turning against him. He knew in his heart that it wasn't really his mother talking, but some illness he didn't understand. Still, it took every ounce of his willpower to walk out the door each morning, never knowing if his mother would greet him with silence or tears when he returned.

After learning from the family doctor that Irene was stricken with Alzheimer's, he hired a neighbor to assist her while he was at work. Her condition worsened over the next few months and before long she required twenty-four-hour care. Bill was forced to place her in a foster home where he hoped the homey environment would comfort her, but he quickly realized she wasn't getting the attention she needed, and he moved her to a nursing home with more intensive care.

I began working for Bill regularly after I returned from college, shortly before he placed Irene in the nursing home. I watched him faithfully visit her over the remaining years of her life. Every Tuesday and Thursday evening after work, Bill would take the bus to Saint Joseph's Nursing Home. Since he worked long days, he often didn't arrive until after regular visiting hours were over. The nurses always nodded him in, as they appreciated the love and devotion he had for his mother. Every Sunday after church, Bill spent the entire afternoon with her. This schedule never changed, even when her condition worsened to the point where she didn't even recognize him.

As our relationship evolved from employer/employee to friendship, Bill turned to my family and me for comfort and support. We opened up our personal lives to each other. I usually talked about how busy I was with my two toddlers, and he invariably talked about Irene and her condition. Progressively, his reports grew worse and worse, from "a little better" to "okay" to "not so well." I sensed his mother's time here on earth was nearing an end.

He asked me if I would like to visit her, but unfortunately I didn't go right away; I was so busy with my own affairs: selling our house, shopping for a new one, volunteering at the church, and participating at a child care cooperative. Time slipped away, and Bill, like a bird on my shoulder, periodically asked, "Shelly, do you think you could come with me sometime soon to visit my mother?" I really wanted to go with him and promised I would check my calendar. Things were so hectic. The children needed me. The church needed me. I was experiencing severe headaches that the doctor told me were due to my being pregnant. Life was so busy, with home shopping and doctor visits and those excruciating headaches.

Through it all, I'd hear the occasional "Shelly, please come with me to visit my mother."

"Soon," I promised. "How about one week from today? We're right in the middle of selling our house."

Exactly one week later, while I was getting ready to deliver Watkins Products, I started spotting blood. Frantic, I phoned the doctor's office for advice, and the nurse assured me, "There is nothing to worry about. Bleeding is quite common. Everything will be fine."

I asked her if I should go to bed or stay off my feet. She told me not to change my routine. If I were going to miscarry, I would miscarry. There was nothing I could do to change it. With great trepidation, I completed packing the orders for Bill.

Later that evening at Bill's house, I sensed that something was seriously wrong with me and decided to postpone our date to visit his mother until I felt better. "Minor female discomfort" was all I said, as I didn't want to upset him with the details of my difficult pregnancy. He was very prone to doting over me, and he had enough on his mind between his mother and his business.

My children spent the day with grandma while I stoically delivered the customers' Watkins products. I was so confident in my ability to deal with the pregnancy that I encouraged my husband to spend the weekend with his brothers in Seattle celebrating multiple birthdays. I promised to call if things got worse.

Sunday morning, I found myself in bed cramping, bleeding, and crying as I waited for John, my husband, to make the three-hour drive home from Seattle. We went immediately to the hospital emergency room, where the doctor tried to locate the baby's heartbeat. There was none! I lay in excruciating pain for hours, pleading for painkillers and verbally attacking every nurse who entered my room.

"I don't do labor," I demanded. "I get epidurals. I don't do this when I am pregnant. Why do I have to do it now?"

Finally, I was wheeled to the ultrasound room where a nurse matter-of-factly informed me that the fetus was dead. Suddenly I felt a gush and the attendant bluntly exclaimed, "Oh, here it is. You've miscarried. It's all over." I sat up to see. She pushed me back down and said, "You don't want to see this."

As she exited the room with my baby wrapped in a towel, she turned and said, "The doctor will be in shortly to perform a D and C, which is a procedure to clean out your insides." (Those really were her exact words!)

There were flowers, cards, meals brought in, and lots of hugs, but no baby. Thanks to two healthy children and a loving husband my life went on. We explained to the children that the baby in mommy's tummy got sick, died, and went to heaven.

Before I knew it, two months went by, and we were at last moved into our much-needed larger home. Life was just beginning to settle down when I heard those familiar words: "Shelly, will you come with me to see my mother?" I was finally able to spend an evening with Bill and his mother.

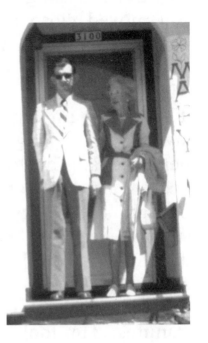

It was a warm August evening when I drove with Bill to Saint Joseph's Nursing Home. He talked nonstop about his mother: how she had changed, how things used to be, how I wouldn't recognize her, and how long it had been since she recognized him. He spoke of her sense of humor, how she loved looking her best, and how stubborn she could be. Bill said the doctors didn't think she would live much longer. He couldn't imagine life without her. In a sense, with her Alzheimer's disease so advanced, she was already gone.

We arrived at Saint Joseph's and Bill led

the way to his mother's room. Our visit was brief; a shriveled shell of a woman lay in bed and stared vacantly at the curtain separating her from her roommate. Her mouth quivered slightly, releasing a senseless, soft muttering. Bill moved close to her, and leaning over he whispered, "Mother, there's someone I want you to see. Do you remember Shelly? Mother? Mother?" Her eyes remained vacant. There was no sign of recognition. She just lay there, rocking, moaning, and pulling at her fingers. The look in Bill's eyes broke my heart. I think my presence must have brought the reality of her condition into perspective for Bill. He fidgeted, looked at his watch, and said, "She's not herself. We should go."

I asked Bill if we could stay for a few more minutes. He looked nervous and upset but agreed. I approached Irene and said, "Mrs. Porter, it's me Shelly. I'm Bill's friend. I work for him."

I gently placed my hand on her forehead and brushed her thin gray hair away from her face. I took her hand in mine, and she stopped rocking. "That's a pretty good kid you have there. He turned out all right. He can be a tough boss, though."

Bill smiled at that. Then I leaned over and whispered in her ear. "Don't worry about Bill. He's going to be just fine. He's a part of my family now, and we'll keep an eye on him for you." I gave her a soft kiss on the forehead and then stepped back so Bill could say his good-bye.

The drive home was mostly quiet and subdued; we both knew her death was not far away. Bill felt a need to apologize. "I'm so sorry. That just wasn't my mother. She's changed so much in the past few months. I wish you could have seen her sooner." Tears came to my eyes and I said, "So do I Bill, so do I. I'm so sorry."

One week later Bill called me; I could barely understand him through the sobbing. "My mother . . . the doctor called . . . it's my mom . . . she's dying . . . can you come now? Will you come with me?"

"I'm on my way," I said.

She was gone by the time we got there. Her body remained atop the bed, eyes open, more vacant than before, cheeks sunken in, and her mouth open as if she tried to utter some last words. Her hair was a disheveled mess and her arthritic hands were clenched. It was a very discomforting sight, and Bill could hardly stand to see her like that. Moving to her bedside, he fell across her, sobbing, "Mother, oh mother."

I felt so awkward being there, just watching, like an intruder standing in the shadows. Bill was draped over her body, tears streaming down his face. I wanted to leave him alone with her, but I couldn't just walk away; he might need me at any moment. I placed my hand on his shoulder to let him know he wasn't alone in this world.

After a few more minutes he was ready to go. During the drive home, Bill was silent except for an occasional stifled sob. I can't remember the exact words of comfort I offered, but they seemed to help as his sobs became fewer and farther between.

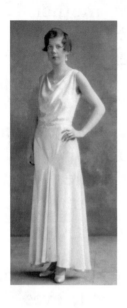

The next day the priest, the nursing facility, and the funeral home helped Bill arrange the funeral. Five days later I stood by Bill's side at the funeral parlor with Irene in a casket for final viewing, but Bill wouldn't approach her. I left him with friends while I walked to the casket. She was wearing a beautiful dress Bill had selected for her. Her hair was neatly styled and the color in her face was restored with makeup. She looked at peace, as if she were only napping — nothing like the way I saw her only five nights before. I knew Bill needed to see her like this before the burial.

I approached him and said, "You really should see your mother." He said, "No, Shelly, I can't. I don't want to remember her like this." I pressed further. "I think it would be a good thing for you to say good-bye one last time." I knew that if Bill viewed her now it would help erase the image of her in that hospital room.

He kept saying "No" and I, in turn, gently persisted. "Bill, trust me. She looks so young and beautiful. Come with me. Come say good-bye." He finally went limp, and I took his hand and led him to the casket. He was amazed how beautiful she looked. "That's how I remember her. Isn't she beautiful? Thank you, Shelly." I watched as he caressed her hands and touched her cheek. He then leaned over and whispered in her ear, "Good-bye."

Bill made it through his mother's death, resumed his daily routine, and went on to become the role model he is today. The Brady family carried on, too; our third daughter, Teressa Amy Nicole, was born May 2, 1990. I learned from Bill that death need not devastate the living. The last thing Irene would have 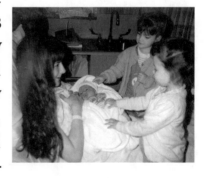 wanted was for Bill to be incapacitated by her death. Instead, her memory continued to motivate and influence Bill's life as he went on to become a great salesman and an inspiration to many. Whenever Bill receives acknowledgement for his achievements, he always humbly replies, "My mother would be so proud."

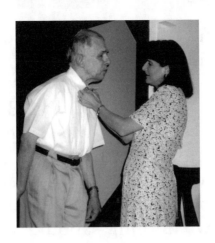

Chapter 7

Be a Team Player

At first glance, watching Bill Porter trek up the steep sidewalks and driveways of his West Portland territory, one sees a solitary man going it alone against the elements. Often it's only Bill and the mailman out there in the rain, sleet, or snow. The mailman is supported by the U.S. Postal Service with its fleet of airplanes, trucks, clerks, and mail sorters; Bill isn't so lucky. Although Watkins, Inc., provides Bill with some support, he is essentially an independent representative who can't count on a substitute to fill in for him when he's sick or when it's raining and the wind is blowing sideways. Over the years, however, Bill has assembled his own team of support personnel that allow him to perform his job as efficiently as the mail carrier (some say more efficiently) in spite of his physical handicaps.

I've known and worked for Bill for more than twenty years and was surprised and a little embarrassed to learn from Tom Hallman's November 1995 feature article in the *Oregonian* that there are members of his team I knew nothing about. Hallman followed Bill on foot to learn exactly how a person with cerebral palsy could accomplish the phenomenal feats that Bill does on a daily basis. He learned the extensive list of players on Bill's team, carefully chosen by Bill over the years, as necessity and situations dictated.

When Irene became ill and was placed in a nursing home, Bill was alone for the first time in his life. He'd never shopped for groceries, prepared meals, or done his own laundry. Irene handled those things while Bill was busy doing what he does best — selling. It didn't take more than a few days for Bill to realize he didn't have the time or physical ability to actually shop, cook, and clean if he intended to service his accounts properly. He quickly put out the word to friends, neighbors, and the congregation at his church that he was hiring for various tasks. Two people from church answered his call. Bill needed one of them to shop, clean the house, and wash his clothes, and the other to keep his yard presentable. Both offered to perform these duties for free. This sounded too much like charity to Bill; he has always insisted on paying people the going wage. I believe that one reason Bill prefers to pay people for their services is because he can then expect a higher level of job performance from everyone he hires.

Bill wasn't a novice employer. Since 1961 he has employed people, including myself, to deliver Watkins products. My association with him began in 1980 when I answered an ad he posted on the Grant High School Job Board. In 1987, I took on other duties for Bill, including housecleaning, laundry, and grocery shopping.

Occasionally, before church or social gatherings, I would button Bill's cuffs or tie his shoelaces for him, never questioning how these tasks were performed when I wasn't around. I must have presumed he had better control of his fingers back then, or someone else magically appeared every day to help him out. Tom Hallman found the latter to be closer to the truth. He followed Bill one morning to the Vintage Plaza Hotel in downtown Portland, where years before Bill had approached the manager to ask for assistance with his buttons and tie. Bill tells the story this way:

"The day after I had my mother placed in a foster home, I didn't know what I'd do.

She was always there for me. She would button my cuffs and collar and put on my tie. I thought about it for a while and then I got an idea. The bus stop downtown where I made my transfer to the West Hills bus was near the Vintage Plaza Hotel. I would carry my tie in my briefcase and ask the manager there if the bellhops could help me."

The manager, Craig Thompson, was happy to accommodate Bill. Every week, Monday through Friday, just after 8:00 A.M., Bill would arrive in the lobby of the hotel, cuffs unbuttoned and tie stashed in his briefcase. Guests and employees came and went but Bill was always there. If it was a busy morning, Bill would patiently wait out of the way until one of the bellhops could assist him. He never waited long, though; they always tried to help him as quickly as they could because they knew he had a full day ahead of him. The employees of the hotel had a good rapport with Bill, too. They all felt they were essentially in the same line of work — pleasing their customers. Bill came to know them all personally; he learned about their birthdays, college applications, marriages, and children.

When Craig Thompson transferred to the Fifth Avenue Suites Hotel a few blocks away, Bill made the switch as well. Craig was delighted to have a familiar face greet him each morning, and Bill quickly made new friends with the staff there. I once asked Bill if it bothered him that he had to ask for help with his tie and buttons.

"It's something I have to do," he replied. "It doesn't bother me at all. The people at the hotel are my friends and they like to help me. I don't look at myself as different from any other person just because I need a little help. It's just part of my daily routine."

The bellhops refused payment for this small service — not even a tip — and, remarkably, Bill accepted the arrangement based on friendship.

After talking with Bill about his dependence on others to complete his dressing, I wondered if under the same circumstances I would have had the courage to ask others for help. I quickly realized that we all need help, we all lack skill of some sort or another. It's just that most of our inabilities aren't so visually evident as Bill's; they may be psychological rather than physical, and, often, we create them ourselves. And, as we all know, some of our self-imposed mental disabilities can be more difficult to overcome than physical ones. All Bill Porter needs is someone to button his cuffs and clip his tie; it's the rest of us who need attitude adjustments, R&R, and pep talks. In my clearest moments, I am able to see Bill Porter as he sees himself and truly say "What disability?"

When *Oregonian* journalist Tom Hallman

approached Bill about writing an article about him, Bill wondered why anyone would want to read about his life. Several years later, he still wonders what all the fuss is about. He's amazed at the letters, gifts, awards, and media attention. It moves him deeply to be told he is a role model, a hero. With humble gratitude he has accepted gifts of money for future medical expenses and retirement. He is touched that businesses, schools, and churches want to hear his story. For example, after hearing Bill and I speak, one company (Primerica Financial Services) sent Bill and the entire Brady family to Disneyland. When asked to comment on all that's happened, he simply responds, "My mother would be so proud. Sales have been very good. And, oh yeah, I got to ride Splash Mountain."

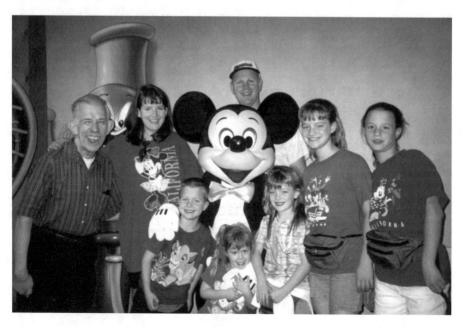

Bill simply doesn't have a clue about the millions of lives he has touched. After the *Oregonian* article, Bill's story was shared in several magazines and news shows. Eventually, ABC's *20/20* got wind of the story. After coming to Portland to film and interview Bill, ABC aired Bill's story, "A Moving Journey," on December 12, 1997. It received the largest viewer response in the history of the program. Thousands of readers faxed, phoned, e-mailed, and wrote, saying how inspired they were by Bill Porter's story.

Over the more than twenty years I've been on Bill's team, many people have told me that I'm an angel for delivering Watkins products for him. I immediately correct them.

"I'm no angel. Bill pays me! I work for him. He's my boss!"

The first time Bill and I shared his story at a business meeting, I tried to explain our employee/employer relationship. Bill jumped right in. "Shelly's an angel." A good-natured argument took place as we went back and forth.

"I'm not an angel, Bill. I work for you," I would say.

Bill, normally quiet, responded with "I couldn't get along without Shelly." I shot right back, "Now that's a bunch of baloney, Bill. You got along for years without me, and if you hadn't hired me in 1980, you would have hired someone else."

Bill replied, "But I did hire you, Shelly. And you are an angel."

I managed to get in the last word. "All right, Bill, that's enough. These people didn't pay good money to bring us all this way to stand here and argue."

At the conclusion of a recent presentation to Callaway Golf in San Diego, I asked Bill if he had any words for the group. Bill replied, "Don't think about your handicaps or problems, think about the things you do have. And then be the best that you can be. That's what I try to do. And when I was too busy or unable to do something myself, I hired someone. I couldn't have sold all those products all these years without help from Shelly and many others. If my story could even touch maybe eleven lives, I would be so glad to have helped those people."

Of course, everyone who heard Bill speak that evening knew that his story has inspired thousands. Since Tom Hallman's article in the *Oregonian* and the *20/20* feature story, Bill's life and mine have been filled with appointments, travel, and speeches. It has been exciting and rewarding beyond my wildest dreams. However, since I am allotted only twenty-four hours per day, I soon felt the quality of my domestic life was in danger of being compromised. How was I going to maintain a successful business life and a healthy and happy family life? (Choosing to have six children didn't make the situation any easier.) In other words, how was I going to have my cake and eat it too? I took a cue from Bill Porter. I discovered I was surrounded by a trusted team of family, friends, and employees to help with my "handicap" of too many high goals and aspirations.

When Bill and I first began traveling to speaking engagements, I haphazardly enlisted the aid of my husband and various babysitters to hold down the fort while I was gone. I felt guilty about leaving the children to my loving husband whose hopes of a round of golf were now completely dashed. For awhile I would call home hourly to make sure everyone was fine. Did you change the diapers? What were your grades on your report card? I love you! See you in two days.

My self-esteem was never higher. My dream of standing on stage with an important message — the message of Bill Porter — was being fulfilled. My heart soared when the audience applauded. I was doing something important and fulfilling. At the same time, I was so worried about my family's well-being that by the time I off-loaded at the Portland International Airport, any good feelings that came from my speeches with Bill were dissipated by my sense of guilt for having left in the first place. If only I could merge my two worlds into one, but it was inconceivable to think that my family would be waiting in the green room after every presentation.

I had a mental handicap that was preventing me from enjoying what should be the happiest days of my life. I was brought up to think that I, the family matriarch, had to do everything myself. Finally, I gave in to a suggestion from Bill. He said, "Do what I did. Hire someone." And I did just that; I hired an occasional housekeeper. Surprisingly, I didn't feel less of a wife or mother for not doing all the household chores myself (not to mention the house is cleaner than ever).

When the requests for presentations by Bill and I reached four per month, I could no longer keep up with the paperwork, the travel arrangements, the billing, and the presentations themselves. I needed another member on my team to handle our bookings in a calm and professional manner. I then learned from a fellow speaker that there are agents who specialize in handling speakers such as Bill and I. They ensure that you are compensated fairly and that all arrangements are in order. Bill and I would then be able to concentrate on putting on a good show. The commission charged is more than made up for by the pressures the agency alleviates.

And so with the aid of family, friends, and a few employees, I am better able to appreciate the time I spend with my family, while the joy I get from traveling to share Bill's story lasts until our next adventure. From Bill, I learned to accept the help of others without feeling less of a person. I also learned that others are just as capable as I am of doing many tasks that I thought only I could do perfectly.

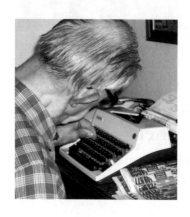

Chapter 8

If It Isn't Broken, Don't Fix It

There is a fine line between disciplined persistence and plain old stubbornness. Bill
walks that line every day of his life. Once he
finds a routine that works, he sticks to it like
glue.

For more than thirty years, Bill has followed a daily regimen like clockwork: up at
4:45, get dressed, eat breakfast, read the
paper, listen to the weather report on the
radio, have his mother help him with his tie
and buttons, collect his briefcase, don his
coat and hat, and head out the door to catch
the 7:20 bus to downtown. Bill then walks
three blocks to transfer to the number 10
bus, which takes him to his sales territory,
the West Hills of Portland, arriving there at
approximately 8:30.

Once in his sales district, he punches a mental time clock and doesn't consider punching out until at least an eight-hour day has been accomplished. All day long Bill walks up and down steep hills, knocking on doors and ringing doorbells; taking a break isn't even considered. But no matter where he is on his route, he stops for lunch at 1:30 P.M. sharp. In the past he liked to be near Saint Thomas More Church for lunch, where he would sit on a bench in the courtyard of the church and eat the lunch that Irene prepared for him. The priests and church secretaries could usually tell what time it was by Bill's arrival and departure. Sometimes Father Dernbach would sit and visit with him for awhile. When his pocket watch read 2:30, it was time to hit the pavement again.

Bill used to call it quits around 6:30, but as the years passed, more women joined the work force and he found fewer people at home during the day. Consequently, his workday stretched into the evening in order to catch customers arriving home from work. Most evenings it would be after 8:30 when he knocked on his last door. When Bill returned home, he'd orchestrate his evening hours as fastidiously as he choreographed his daylight hours. First, he sat in his easy chair, kicked off his shoes, and looked over his orders while his mother prepared dinner. Irene loved hearing every detail of Bill's day: who placed an order, who didn't and why, even if the knots on his shoelaces lasted all day. During dinner he'd usually listen to a radio talk show or sports event. Finally, he'd soak in a hot bath to try to get the kinks out of his back and sore muscles before climbing into bed by 11:00.

When his mother was no longer in their home to help Bill put the finishing touches on his sales attire, he added two stops to his morning ritual. First he'd stop at the shoe-shine shop where he'd have his shoes shined and laces tightened, and then on to the Fifth Avenue Suites for help with his buttons and tie. In the evenings, Bill would turn the radio on for company and put two frozen TV dinners in the oven. When special errands had to be run, such as a haircut or shopping, Bill worked longer days to justify the time off.

When I started working for him as a teenager, I learned quickly that Bill likes things the way they are. I wasn't to move his furniture around or reorganize his knick-knacks. Once, while cleaning Bill's house, I folded and hung his bath towels the wrong way; he called me on the phone asking me if I was feeling all right. I said I felt fine. He was worried I might be ill because I had put the towels out improperly. I apologized and never got it wrong again!

When Watkins began encouraging sales representatives to consider multi-level marketing strategies, Bill wasn't interested; it didn't fit his style of selling. He thought it was fine that more than eighty thousand Watkins distributors built their businesses in that manner, but at that time Bill didn't want to spend his time and energy directing a "down-line." ("Down-line" refers to the customers and other sales people who work with a salesperson in a network.)

Years ago, Bill didn't have an answering machine, a VCR, a microwave, cable television, or a cordless phone. He still wouldn't if well-wishers hadn't given him all those things as gifts. Before they arrived on his front doorstep, I clearly remember Bill's outspokenness about modern gadgets.

"What use is an answering machine? I've gotten along for half a century just fine without owning one. If someone wants to reach me when I'm out, they'll keep trying if it's important enough. Why would I want to tie myself to a machine that makes me feel obligated to get back to someone I might not have wanted to talk to in the first place? Unless, of course, someone is calling to buy something from me."

Those calls are pretty rare because he stays on top of his customers' needs.

The VCR is still a mystery to Bill. It comes in handy when friends want to view the videotape of his appearance on ABC's *20/20*, a recent speaking engagement, or an awards ceremony. But he usually asks the guest to operate the VCR. Bill and I still chuckle about the time he complained that the VCR wasn't working; he told me he stuck in a tape and nothing happened. Thank goodness nothing happened — he'd inserted a cassette tape!

I was excited when Bill received a microwave as a gift. I thought it would cut down on food preparation time and ensure that he ate better, but he refused to touch it for three weeks. He spent another two weeks experimenting with opening and closing it. Finally, after many practice sessions, Bill felt comfortable warming one of his frozen dinners in the microwave, but since he eats two frozen dinners at his evening meal he still uses his conventional oven for one of them. I showed him how two dinners would fit in the microwave, but no amount of logic or coaxing convinced him to prepare his meals this way. There is something about the anticipation Bill feels while waiting the thirty to forty minutes it takes for a TV dinner to warm in the oven. It gives him time to sit down, take off his shoes, read the paper, and relax while the aroma of dinner fills the air. Perhaps it reminds him of the good old days when Irene made home-cooked meals.

Cable television was one of Bill's favorite gifts. Always an avid sports fan, he was now able to watch the Portland Trailblazers on

Blazer Cable. Other than sports broadcasts, though, Bill rarely watches television. In fact, he prefers to watch games with the television volume turned down and the radio blaring. Having been a sports journalist in high school, Bill relates to the sports announcer whose goal is to paint a picture in the listener's mind.

The cordless phone is one modern gadget Bill adapted to immediately. Before this handy invention, Bill used to spend hours each month typing me a grocery list so I could do his shopping. Now, he walks around the kitchen, opens cupboards, and recites his needs to me via the cordless phone. This saves him time and ensures that he doesn't forget necessary items as he opens cupboard after cupboard. Once Bill was especially excited because he was calling me from his backyard while he described his plants and shrubs. He rarely gabs on the phone, though. In spite of its convenience, it's still just a novelty to Bill. To him, the phone is mostly a business tool that greatly increases sales and allows him to better serve his accounts.

Several people and companies attempted to give Bill a computer as a gift. One kind lady went so far as to set one up in Bill's house. Bill experimented with it, but all that he got out of it when he typed his name was "BBBBB" and "Poooorrtterr." That was the end of that. No way was he replacing his manual typewriter with a computer. He just laughed when I assured him that a computer would simplify his record keeping. "No it won't," he said, "because I won't have one of those contraptions in my home."

Bill may be a lot wiser than many of us when it comes to the use of high-tech gadgets. When I count the hours I've spent at the computer "saving time" only to have the program crash, I know in my heart that Bill may be the smart one to stick with pecking away at the keys on his manual typewriter. I've learned from Bill that a simple, gadget-free life can sometimes be a better one. He doesn't have to worry about answering e-mails or taping mindless television shows. He isn't constantly updating his computer and the software needed to run it. He is busy living life, meeting people one on one, face to face, and not carrying on conversations out in cyberspace. He takes the time to smell the roses or at least the dinner cooking. Why fix what isn't broken?

Every time someone in my family physically injures themselves, I tell a story Bill told me about the time he took a terrible spill on the sidewalk in front of a customer's house.

"I tripped and fell, landing on my chin," he states matter-of-factly. "Blood was everywhere. One of my customers drove me to the hospital and stayed by my side until the doctor could see me. I ended up with seven stitches. She wanted to drive me home afterwards so I could rest, but I wasn't finished with my selling day. I told her I'd rather be driven back to my territory."

And sure enough, Bill finished his eight-hour day, bandaged chin and all, staying a little longer than usual to make up for the time he spent at the hospital.

The story would have ended much differently if the same accident had happened to me. I would have gone home to bed, called my husband on the cordless, moaned that I was in too much pain to cook, and asked him to bring home a pizza. I've been known to do that after stubbing my toe or breaking a fingernail. Seven stitches could possibly buy me a week in bed. Then, I'd get out of bed only to use the restroom, get popcorn refills, and answer e-mails.

I've seen Bill confined to bed on only two occasions, and to see my unstoppable friend physically "broken" is heart wrenching. For the first fourteen years I knew him, Bill never took a day off from work. Nothing kept him home, not a cold, flu, arthritis, not even his intense migraine headaches. But after years of pounding the pavement with an excruciatingly painful back condition, Bill finally sought help from a doctor. After trying everything from oral medication to cortisone shots to physical therapy, his doctor said back surgery was the only way to stop the pain. He also let Bill know that there was the very real possibility he may not be able to walk again if the surgery wasn't successful. Unwilling to take such a risk, Bill put off the surgery. The days turned into weeks, weeks into months, months into years. Eventually the pain became so intense it outweighed the risks of surgery and Bill agreed to the operation.

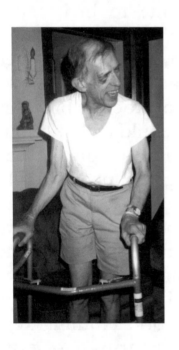

The surgery was postponed until after the 1993 holiday season because Bill wanted to conclude the year with top sales honors. Unfortunately, he had cancelled his health insurance a few years prior because he couldn't afford the premiums. To make matters worse, he had decided a few years back to take out a second mortgage on his paid-for house for some much-needed improvement projects. In 1990, he consolidated all his outstanding debt into one equity loan with a high interest loan company (i.e., loan shark) that solicited his business over the phone. The telemarketer convinced Bill it would make things easier to pool his financial obligations and only have one check to write. Unfortunately, the high interest on the new loan didn't leave him enough money to pay his property taxes, and so now he faced the real possibility of losing his home to the loan company or to the county for unpaid taxes.

Meanwhile, the back operation was scheduled for the end of January 1994. Bill's life was falling to pieces, physically and financially. One afternoon he swallowed his pride and told me of his dilemma. Here he was having back surgery, which might put an abrupt end to his only source of income — door-to-door sales. He didn't know if he would ever walk again, let alone make a living. To top it off, he didn't know if he would own a home to rehabilitate himself in.

My husband John and I had an immediate family meeting. We had recently refinanced our home to take advantage of lower interest rates, and, like Bill, we set aside extra money in the loan package for some home projects, including city-mandated sewer improvements. The day before my conversation with Bill, we had made an early payment of four thousand dollars to the city, leaving us with little cash with which to help Bill. What if we called the sewer office to get that check back and used the money instead as a down payment for the purchase of Bill's house? He could rent it from us for far less money than he was making in loan payments each month.

We approached Bill with our proposal. Before we could say more than a few words, he told us he had been thinking along the same lines. The next few days were a blur as we made phone calls, managed to get our check back, filled out dozens of documents, and finally secured the money to pay off Bill's high-interest loan, past-due property taxes, and other assorted debts. We then turned around and rented the house to Bill for much less than he had been paying for the loan.

It was frightening for us at the time to take on the financial risk of another mortgage because in 1994 we added child number four, Kevin Patrick, for a grand total of six mouths to feed. We were stretched to our financial limits. But as long as Bill made his portion, we could survive. If he was unable to work after his back surgery, I was prepared to work part-time at McDonald's, because in our hearts we felt good about what had transpired for two reasons: most importantly, it was a way to help our friend Bill, and, of course, it would be a good long-term investment for us.

Bill's surgery did go very well. The doctor ordered bed rest and restricted the use of stairs. Bill ignored the doctor's orders and rested only when pain forced him to. Remarkably, his strength returned rapidly, and after only two months Bill was anxious to reconnect with his Watkins accounts.

He began by selling over the telephone, and his loyal client base gladly placed their orders. (My fantasy of a two-month vacation from Watkins deliveries flew out the window.) Bill was happy to just be selling again but complained that he dearly missed door-to-door sales. On the 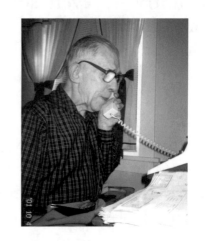 telephone, he found he "traveled" too quickly through his territory, missing out on the subtle delights involved in meeting one-on-one with his customers. No one believed it was possible, but in May 1994, only four months after his surgery, Bill was back at it, pounding the pavement. The doctors were truly amazed that anyone could be up and about so quickly, let alone someone with cerebral palsy. Soon, his back surgery and time off were a distant memory, and it was back to business for Bill and Shelly, and business was good.

The year 1997 brought new adventures for Bill and myself. The *Oregonian* article, just a little more than a year old, was still attracting new customers and media attention. ABC's *20/20* came out to film Bill's story, with plans to air it later in the year to more than twenty million viewers. Companies all over the country — even some from abroad — clamored for us to tell Bill's inspiring story at their conventions. Hollywood producers and actors expressed interest in making a movie of Bill's life. Book publishers called to see if I was interested in writing a book about him. Then, exactly one week after the *20/20* piece was filmed in late July, Bill stepped off the curb in front of his house and was sideswiped by a distracted driver. One split second changed Bill's life and mine forever.

Like victims of an earthquake remembering where they were when the big one hit, I remember Bill's accident and the events leading up to it as if they happened yesterday. The week started out insanely for me. I promised to help a friend with her daughter's wedding, a Japanese exchange student was arriving to stay with us, and we were busy packing for our annual family camping trip. On top of all this, I was watching two children for a friend, my house was a mess, and because of the trip I needed to deliver the Watkins products a couple of days early.

I headed to the grocery store with seven children. We did Bill's shopping and drove to his house to put away the groceries and clean. Michelle changed the sheets. Katrina scrubbed the bathroom. Tessa and Joey (a friend's son) dusted everything. Kevin and

Kelsey (friend's daughter) played with the baby (Erica, our fifth). I supervised, hoping to get things cleaned as quickly as possible because Bill was due home around 2:30, when he would give me the exact directions for the deliveries.

Rarely did I ask Bill to modify delivery days; remember, he doesn't like change! Years of friendship softened him somewhat, and if a real need presented itself, Bill could be swayed a little. So knowing Bill usually typed the directions to the houses on Tuesdays, I asked him if he could dictate them to me when I came over to clean on Monday. (This would take about half an hour as opposed to the thirteen hours Bill normally spends typing directions.) He told me he had personal errands to run on Monday and would be home sometime after noon, at the latest 2:30. I told him I'd be at his house by 1:00, certain he'd be back no later than 1:30 as he always likes to be home when I am there.

One-thirty came and went. I was surprised, but figured he'd be home by 2:30 for sure. When 2:30 came and went, knowing how punctual he always is, I began to worry. Where could he be? By 3:00 we were finished cleaning and still no Bill. I began to panic. *Why hasn't he called? What on earth was the problem? A missed bus connection, a new customer? What? He's never late without calling.* I sent the children out to the back yard to play because they were getting restless, and I didn't want them to mess up the house.

A car pulled up and I ran to the door. It was my in-laws, Deborah and Gary Wood; Bill had hired them to do his yard work. They had come to drop off a receipt for a garden hose.

No, they hadn't seen Bill. They had worked in the yard that morning, but Bill had already left to run errands. While Gary, Deborah, and I stood on the porch talking about where Bill could be, a stranger approached the house. From here on out, everything seemed to happen in slow motion. The words that came out of the stranger's mouth sounded like a 45-rpm record played at 33 rpm. Everything was surreal, as if I was dreaming, except this dream was quickly turning into a nightmare.

"Bill was hit by a car this morning," the stranger said.

A stunned silence followed. Finally, I was able to activate my vocal chords.

"Is he okay? What happened? Do you know where he is? Who hit him? Is he badly injured?"

When I finally shut up long enough to hear an answer, the stranger said, "An ambulance took Bill away. His forehead was cut, and he was walking around and arguing with the ambulance driver about him not needing to go to the hospital. They finally convinced him to get into the ambulance." The stranger didn't know where they took Bill. I later found out that he was Bill's neighbor.

After thanking him, I went into the house, opened the phone book to the yellow pages, and proceeded to call hospital after hospital. Three phone calls in a row yielded no patient by the name of Bill Porter. At last, on my fourth attempt, Emanuel Hospital confirmed that a William Douglas Porter was admitted to the emergency room earlier in the day, and was transferred to the X-ray department. She wasn't sure where he was at the time. I ended the conversation and quickly loaded seven restless children into my van. Emanuel Hospital was only seven short minutes away.

Once there, I learned the gash on Bill's head required stitches, but his X ray indicated no other problems. However, because Bill appeared disoriented they felt it necessary to refer him to social services.

"Why didn't someone call me?" I wanted to know. Meanwhile, the children made the best of the situation by sliding down banisters and jumping on the sofas in the lobby; I attempted to contact social services and, of course, an answering machine was the only response I got. Upset because I didn't know what happened to Bill, I snapped at the children to "sit still." If he was discharged, then where is he? Why didn't he go home? I pleaded with the hospital receptionist to please try to reach the social service agent for me. Within minutes, the agent answered the page and I asked her what happened to Bill. She said she tried to convince him to go home and rest as he had taken quite a tumble. She offered to get him a cab. He'd refused, saying that it was only a few stitches and he had to finish some errands. *Oh no,* I thought, *there he goes again.* "If it isn't completely broken, why fix it?"

Since there was nothing else to accomplish at the hospital, I headed home with seven very hungry and cranky children. Naturally, I swung by Bill's in the hope that he would be there; no such luck. I tried to convince myself that he lost track of time after his accident, but realized that wasn't possible; this is Bill we're dealing with, after all. Surely he would remember his dear friend Shelly, and how worried sick she would be.

At 6:00 the phone rang. It was Bill.

"Where are you? Why haven't you called?" I asked.

His voice was slurred and it was extremely difficult to decipher his words. "I was hit by a car," he said.

"I know. I've been trying to find you. Where are you?" I demanded.

"I'm at Providence Hospital. I left my house this morning to run my errands downtown. I stepped onto the street and the next thing I knew there was a car coming at me and I went stumbling to the ground. The driver pulled out to make a left turn. He says he didn't see me because the sun was in his eyes. What kind of excuse is that?"

He sounded angry. I tried to calm him. "It was an accident, Bill. The driver must feel terrible. I wouldn't want to be in either one of your shoes. So, did he actually hit you?"

"I don't know. I think so. There were two people standing at the bus stop. One of them says he hit me. The other thinks he might have stopped just before hitting me and that it startled me and I fell. I'm pretty banged up for just a fall."

"I heard you got stitches. What else is wrong? Why are you in the hospital? Why didn't you come home? Why didn't you call?"

"The ambulance insisted on taking me to the hospital. I thought it was a waste of time. They stitched up my head and sent me for X rays because my leg and back hurt. When they told me my X rays were clear, I figured it was time to go. Some social service agent wanted me to go home. I told her I was fine and I left."

"Why didn't you go home, Bill? Are you in pain?"

"Of course I'm in pain, but what else is new? Why should I go home for pain when there are things to be done?"

There was no use arguing. What I wanted to know was why Bill was calling from another hospital. He continued.

"I left the hospital and started my errands. I went to the allergy clinic and the bank. Each step got more and more painful. Soon I couldn't go on. I found myself collapsed on the sidewalk in excruciating pain. It felt like knives were stabbing my hips. A passerby called an ambulance. I didn't argue this time. They brought me to Providence Hospital, and they are taking me in for more X rays soon."

I told Bill I was so grateful he called and that he was okay for the most part. He cut off my ramblings to tell me the real reason he called was to give me the delivery directions! Lo and behold, he proceeded with house number one: "Go out Dosch Park Road; take a right on Bridlemile Lane. . . ." What was I to do but write them down? He continued until I heard the nurse in the background saying, "Mr. Porter, we really need to wheel you to X-ray now." I smiled to myself as he said good-bye, promising to call me back with the rest of the directions as soon as he was back in his room.

The next phone call from Bill informed me of his X-ray results: he had fractured his hip in the accident. The break was in such an awkward spot that it didn't surprise the

130

X-ray technician that the other hospital had missed it. The doctor would be performing surgery shortly, so Bill had to quickly recite the rest of the delivery directions. The pain medications slurred his voice to the point where I could barely understand him. Fortunately, I had been delivering for him long enough that I was familiar with the area and the clients. I assured Bill I would not get lost and that all of his Watkins products would be delivered properly and promptly.

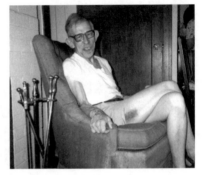

The next two months would prove to be the most challenging in Bill's life since the death of his mother. He arrived home from the hospital one week later, battered and bruised but in good spirits. Once again he was given strict orders to use his walker and stay off of the stairs. Social services brought him a portable commode to discourage him from using the upstairs bathroom.

This time he didn't heal as quickly as he did after back surgery. Two days after arriving home, he suffered a terrible setback. Bill called me saying he felt dizzy and nauseous. I had been at his house only two hours earlier to take pictures of his injuries — a black eye and badly bruised legs — and joking about making a poster that read, "You should see what I did to the other guy!"

I sped back to Bill's and helped him get to bed. We both figured he needed rest. Shortly after I returned home, Bill's neighbor called.

"Bill is in trouble," he said. "Can you please come back? I can't find my key to his house."

By the time I got there, Bill was vomiting and his chest was tight. He was dizzy and pale. It really scared me to see him looking that way. I called 911 and an ambulance took him back to the hospital. I locked up his house, went home, and waited to hear from the doctors.

The next six weeks were a blur. Bill's equilibrium was so poor he wasn't able to walk down the hospital corridor. The hospital staff felt he shouldn't go home anytime soon; they wanted him to spend time at an adult-care facility where he could have twenty-four-hour attention and intense physical therapy. Bill was adamantly opposed to the idea. He wanted to know, "Why can't someone stay with me at my house? Why can't a nurse visit me for therapy twice a week like the hospital said originally?"

I explained that we were all worried about his dizziness, about the risk of falling down if he were home alone, and about the danger of re-injuring his hip. At a care facility, he would receive physical therapy twice a day

132

verses two times a week at home. He'd get well that much faster. I wished I could help him around the clock, but I was scheduled to be out of town and I had my children to look after. I was glad to come over often, but he needed much more than I could give him.

"Please," I begged him. "I would worry much less about you if you stayed in the hands of professionals." Furthermore, Medicare paid almost all the cost of an adult-care facility stay, but would cover very little or none of the cost of at-home care.

After much pleading, Bill reluctantly agreed to stay at the facility. The move almost broke his spirit; he retreated inside himself, as if the world had given up hope on him. No amount of humor seemed to change his attitude. From Bill's point of view, it must have appeared that the establishment finally had him where they wanted him his entire life — in an institution. From our perspective, nothing could be farther from the truth; we wanted him out of the facility as soon as possible. We wanted him well and out here with us, inspiring us as he always has.

I can't remember when things turned around. After many weeks, Bill slowly climbed out of his shell. He stopped complaining "I don't belong here" and "I know I'll never see my front porch again" and started concentrating on regaining his strength. Exactly one day before his sixty-fifth birthday, he received the best present ever: a ride home! His condition was greatly improved and it looked like things might get back to normal.

One month later, Bill felt he was ready to reclaim his territory in person. I remember the wet day in October when I worried about every step, every curb, and every passing car. That evening I called Bill to ask how it went. He sounded very different; there was no spunk or verve in his voice. Words were uttered from Bill's lips that I never thought I'd hear. "I can't do it, Shelly. I tried, but I just can't."

Bill told me what happened that day: "I took the bus to my territory and started walking. Each step became more and more painful until I finally had to sit down on the curb and rest. Before the day was half through, I realized my door-to-door days were over. It took every ounce of strength I had just to make it back to the bus stop. I can't walk my route anymore. I don't know what I'm going to do."

I couldn't sleep that night thinking about what appeared to be my friend's broken spirit. How would this problem be resolved, I wondered? I didn't have to wonder too long, though, because the next morning Bill called with an idea:

"I've made up my mind, Shelly. I'll sell over the phone. I did it three years ago when my back went out and I can do it again."

And Bill Porter did just that! I can attest to the fact that he was every bit as successful, if not more, selling over the phone as he was selling door-to-door. I made his deliveries and he sold so many Watkins products that I had to enlist John and our children to help with deliveries.

By the time ABC's *20/20* segment on Bill aired on December 12, 1997, just five months after his accident, Bill was back to his old self. Most of his successful routines were reinstituted. If something worked in the past, Bill didn't see any need to change it. If change was forced upon him, like a broken hip or back, he learned to adapt his behavior, but only slightly.

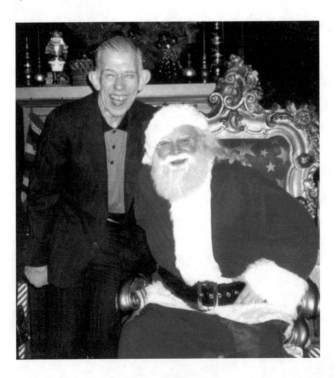

Stubborn determination keeps Bill focused and on track. I remember him lamenting that his favorite team was playing on a Saturday afternoon and how he would have to miss the game because it was during "callbacks." I reminded him he was his own boss, and he could rearrange his hours, watch the game, and do "callbacks" later. He looked at me like I was crazy. I should have known better than to try to help Bill Porter fix something that wasn't broken.

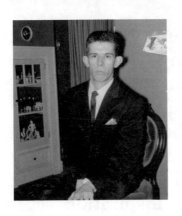

Chapter 9

There Are No Obstacles

The first speaking engagement Bill and I contracted for was titled *Overcoming Obstacles: The Bill Porter Story.* I wanted to prepare fully for the occasion, so with notebook in hand, I asked Bill a few questions. "Bill, I want you to tell me all your obstacles."

After a long silence, I looked up from my notebook to see Bill staring at me. I repeated the question.

"Shelly," Bill stated emphatically, "how many times do I have to tell you and everyone else? I don't have any obstacles. Ask me another question."

We played this cat-and-mouse game for fifteen minutes, with me cleverly rephrasing the question to trick the answer I wanted out of Bill: cerebral palsy, a lack of muscle coordination, an aching back, a speech impediment. I wasn't having any luck; Bill wouldn't play the game with me. He sincerely believes he doesn't have any obstacles of any kind.

I knew audiences admired Bill because he overcame major obstacles in his life, and I wanted to satisfy them. They thought of him as a hero, an inspiration, a man who overcame tremendous odds. After learning from Bill's example, my hope was that audience members with obstacles would be encouraged to overcome them.

However, Bill's stubbornness forced me to change my approach to the speech. Instead of talking about how Bill overcame his obstacles, I was forced to speak about Bill's "perceived" lack of obstacles. The word "obstacle" simply doesn't exist in Bill's vocabulary. He understands an obstacle to be something that totally blocks one from reaching a destination or goal, but the fact of the matter is, Bill never encounters "obstacles" because he always reaches his goal, whether it be a physical location or a sales quota. He is simply unstoppable.

When I was a child, my parents said I could be anything I wanted, the President of the United States or an Olympic swimmer. While I believed they were sincere, I never really took them too seriously; I felt the odds were extremely slim that either could actually happen. I appreciated their confidence in me, but I set my sights on what I considered more realistic, attainable goals such as a college education, a large, loving family, and a rewarding career. (In light of recent presidencies and elections, who really wants to be President of the United States, anyway?)

On the other hand, the opposite is true with Bill. He can quote verbatim what his mother said to him when he was eight years old: "Bill, you can accomplish anything you want, if you just set your mind to it." Bill believed his mother whole-heartedly. I see this positive attitude in Bill's approach to every stumbling block (not obstacle, mind you) he encounters. The following story is a typical example.

A few years ago, an especially cold and icy storm dropped out of Alaska onto the streets of Portland. Bill heard about the storm from the television weather forecasters. Being the complete optimist, however, he figured the forecasters were overestimating its strength. Bill puts a positive spin on weather forecasts in the summertime as well. When the forecasters predict highs in the nineties, he tells me, "I think cool." The weather is very important to Bill because it determines what he wears and whether he should carry an overcoat or an umbrella. On this particular stormy day, Bill dressed appropriately and made his scheduled rounds. Every customer he encountered told him he should call it a day and head for home before the freezing rain started. Bill thought it was a perfect day for door-to-door sales because, as he says, "When the weather gets really nasty, more customers are home."

Finally, after he exceeded his daily quota, he was ready to head home. Unfortunately, Bill didn't outguess the weatherman this time; the buses had stopped running due to the storm and Bill had to hitchhike home. Not only was it bitterly cold and wet, the roads were dangerously slick. By the time he reached the steep driveway leading to his front door, it had frozen into a sheet of black ice as slippery as an ice skating rink. Bill tried again and again to get up his driveway, but he kept falling down. His shoes couldn't get any traction. After several painful falls, he got down on all fours, crawled to his front door, turned the key, stepped inside, and at last proceeded to prepare his dinner while he watched the weather forecast for the next day.

The image of Bill crawling up his driveway on all fours is forever etched in my mind. When I scolded him for not calling for help, he said, "What's the big deal? Nobody could have made it up that driveway without getting down on all fours."

Another example of Bill's refusal to submit to obstacles takes place every evening after he finishes dinner. As I mentioned in an earlier chapter, Bill is wise enough to hire employees when the job at hand is too time-consuming or too difficult for his physical abilities. For instance, I deliver customer's orders for him in my car because he doesn't drive; a gardener keeps his yard neat because it takes him too much time and effort; a housekeeper keeps Bill's home neat and well-stocked with his favorite foods (mostly frozen). I have been Bill's housekeeper for fifteen years and now my children help perform the task.

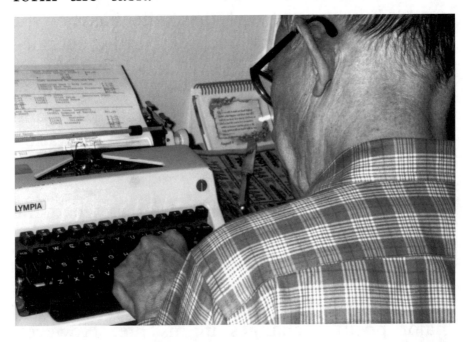

However, even though Bill is familiar with the benefits of employing assistants, I can't convince him to hire a secretary to type his orders. It just pains me to watch him peck away with one finger. Even a mediocre typist could prepare his orders in a matter of minutes. Bill spends hours pecking away, insists on doing all his own typing, and often types superfluous special delivery instructions with each order. *Go down driveway. Open the gate. Leave the package by the back door. Close the gate behind you.* I don't need such detailed instructions and told him so, but he continues to add them anyway.

After the *Oregonian* article appeared, which included a vivid description of Bill's poor typing skills, multiple offers came in for free typing services from professional typists. Bill wouldn't accept any of them; he has to type all orders to ensure accuracy. And actually, Bill seems to enjoy himself as he finger-types each order. This is just another example of Bill turning an obstacle as painstaking and tedious as typing into a form of relaxation where he can reflect on his day and plan out the next.

The following incident temporarily had me believing that Bill's optimistic approach to obstacles was coming to an end. Bill and I credit Tom Hallman's article in the *Oregonian*, "Life of a Salesman," with creating major positive changes in his life. However, very few people know that when the article first appeared on Sunday, November 27, 1995, Bill was extremely upset by it. Personally, I was ecstatic that so many people were learning about my noble and brave friend Bill Porter. Sure, I was a little worried that the detailed description of Bill's handicaps might initially hurt Bill's feelings, but not to the extreme that it did.

When I called him the morning the article came out, he was fit to be tied. He believed he hadn't been treated fairly. He felt the article portrayed him as a freak. The reporter's use of the word "twisted" to describe his body was what irked Bill the most. Keep in mind that Bill Porter is, for good reason, a very proud man. He is a dignified and gracious human being who doesn't see himself as suffering from the physical symptoms associated with cerebral palsy.

I spent the next hour-and-a-half explaining to Bill that Tom Hallman's article was very well written.

"Tom picked the word 'twisted,' " I gently said, "because he needed to paint a picture with words and to aid readers of the article in understanding what cerebral palsy is and the physical limitations that often accompany the disease."

Bill retorted, "My friends and customers don't see me that way. They don't think my body is twisted. Why did he have to pick that word?"

I had never seen Bill so upset in all the years I'd known him. My belief in Bill's ability to overcome all obstacles appeared to fly out the window. I couldn't calm him down. Furthermore, he was annoyed by the vivid description of his nightstand. Mr. Hallman described it as "littered with medications for a body that was in constant pain."

"I am not in constant pain," Bill exclaimed.

"But you are in constant pain," I said. "Step away from yourself for a minute. You have migraines at least two days a week. Your arthritis flares up and your back aches on almost a daily basis. The rest of the world, including doctors, calls that constant pain."

After a few days went by, Bill was still hurt and bitter about the *Oregonian* article. Tom Hallman was very concerned about Bill's response; he expected the exact opposite reaction. He truly has the greatest respect and admiration for Bill, and he asked me if I could speak to Bill and straighten out the misunderstanding. He wanted Bill to realize that his intentions were honorable. He simply wanted the readers of the article to comprehend the full extent of Bill's physical condition so they could more fully appreciate Bill's greatness. The situation was a catch-22: Bill doesn't think he has physical limitations or obstacles, and, being an excellent journalist, Mr. Hallman was obligated to portray the facts accurately, and the fact of the matter is . . . Bill Porter has cerebral palsy.

It wasn't until Bill learned that more than seven hundred readers wrote, e-mailed, or phoned the *Oregonian* wanting to become his customers that Bill finally began to see things differently. "Tom really didn't mean any harm," he stated later. Bill was pleasantly overwhelmed with the arduous task of typing up all those new orders with one finger. He soon broke all existing sales records for Watkins products in the Pacific Northwest. "I guess my back does hurt once in a while," he later admitted.

Most recently, serious health problems have forced Bill to curtail travel by airplane. It wasn't easy for him to admit that there was an obstacle that could best him. Fortunately, my husband and I found innovative, high-tech solutions to the problem.

The discovery that flying wasn't healthy for Bill couldn't have come at a worse time in our busy speaking schedule. We were booked solid for engagements at Amway, Watkins, Disney, Nike, and other companies. We were definitely on a roll. Bill enjoyed the luxurious accommodations, and I thrived on the opportunity to travel and speak.

Then it happened — Bill couldn't catch his breath during a flight to Atlanta as I slept soundly next to him. Bill thought that death wasn't far away. Of course, he didn't bother to nudge me and let me assist him. He made it through his state of panic with the aid of an inhaler, but the incident was incredibly frightening for Bill.

This shortness of breath wasn't new to him; he often experienced it after walking a few blocks. But after resting momentarily and using an inhaler, he was always able to catch his breath and continue. Bill called them "breathing episodes" (in other words, "no big deal"). The doctors believed the shortness of breath was due to progressive, fibrotic lung disease. This ailment originated from an acid-reflux condition, whereby stomach acids cause scarring of the lung tissue. In layman's terms, Bill's lungs weren't capable of processing the oxygen his body needed. The poor air quality on long airplane flights exacerbated the situation.

To compound the problem, Bill began to experience "panic attacks." They occurred whenever he felt he was in a situation where he might lose his breath. These attacks caused Bill's lungs to hyperventilate, thereby triggering a "breathing episode." Bill went through a tug-of-war over whether to continue traveling or give in to his illness and stay near the safety of home. Despite being the brave man who he is, he took one more flight to the East Coast and then called it quits; no more air travel.

Personally, I was devastated by Bill's refusal to travel by plane. I pictured my speaking career coming to an abrupt halt. I thought, *Who wants Shelly without Bill?* Prior to putting the suitcase in the attic, I did some brainstorming with my computer-literate husband. John saw no reason why we couldn't use the latest advances in digital photography and the Internet to "virtually" present Bill on stage with me. Now, when Bill can't be present, I keep a live telephone connection with him while I'm on stage. This way Bill and I can banter back and forth. Bill went along with the program because he knew how much I love public speaking and he loves the publicity, which translates into increased sales.

The presentations, with live audio and/or video feeds to Bill, have gone extremely well. The audience's response to Bill's "virtual" presence has been equal to the responses we received when he was on stage with me.

At the end of most presentations, I ask the audience what they feel is the greatest obstacle Bill overcame. The responses run the gamut: cerebral palsy, back surgery, declining health, death of his mother, inability to drive. The list goes on. I sometimes write these obstacles on a large chalkboard as they are spoken. Then turning to Bill on live video or by telephone, I go down the list: "Was cerebral palsy an obstacle? Was your mother's death an obstacle?" With unwavering conviction, he dismisses each so-called "obstacle" one by one. "I don't believe I have any obstacles at all," he says time and again.

★ ★ ★

The number of people inspired by Bill Porter's life story astounds me. Incredibly, many of these people only know of him from the twenty-minute segment on *20/20* or the *Oregonian* newspaper article. Since I've been an employee and friend of Bill's for many years, it's only natural that he has inspired me. Nearly every day I have watched him routinely conquer greater obstacles than I have faced in my entire life.

Nonetheless, I have struggled with personal obstacles that, at times, have made me feel inadequate and frustrated with myself. Experiences in my youth, for example, affected my attitude towards money and material wealth. When I was twelve years old, my family moved from Portland to Kauai, a small island in Hawaii. My parents moved there for employment that never materialized, and consequently we learned to make do with what little money we had. Out of necessity, my mother learned to bake bread from scratch and grow much of our food in a garden. We hung our laundry in the sun to save electricity. Graciously, we accepted gifts of tropical fruit from friends and neighbors who knew the gifts were much appreciated.

Attire on the islands is much more casual than on the mainland, but we dressed casually because we had no choice. The money simply wasn't available to replace our plastic flip-flops when they became thin and chewed up. In spite of this, I joked about running around in my bare feet like a native child, all the time aware of the endless array of spiffy shoes lining the department store shelves in Honolulu and on the mainland. After all, I was a teenage *houle* (Hawaiian for Caucasian) from the mainland who, at times, longed for a more comfortable lifestyle. Although I cherish my years living on Kauai, I know that's where I adopted a reluctance to spend money that has caused some strife in my marriage over the years.

After the birth of our first child, John and I decided it was time for me to quit my job so I could be a full-time homemaker. It meant changing our lifestyle as we made the shift from two incomes to one. It was a frightening time, but it felt right for us. We scrimped and saved to make house payments on our first home and pay back our school loans. We tightened our belts and took a gigantic leap of faith.

Like my mother on Kauai, I went into survival mode, but instead of raising a garden and baking my own bread, I became an expert at clipping coupons and finding sales. A friend introduced me to thrift stores and garage sales. Before I knew it, my calendar was full: Friday mornings — garage sales, before anyone got there; Saturday afternoons — garage sales, when people wanted to get rid of their stuff at half price; Tuesday — thrift stores, when the "new" used merchandise was put out; Wednesday night — groceries, when the meat and dairy section were marked half-price just prior to the expiration date.

Wherever there was a bargain, I could sniff it out. Intuitively, I knew when to step on the brakes and turn for a sale. I developed a reputation as the "thrift queen," and I was proud of it. I felt that I enabled us to live beyond our means because of my keen eye for bargains. When someone complimented me one time on a new outfit, I proudly responded, "I got this suit at the Value Village for just $1.98, and the shoes were only 99 cents." When company came over, it was always an opportunity for me to "show and tell" my latest findings, from furnishings to closets full of clearance items. I was well prepared for upcoming birthday parties, showers, or weddings.

My husband appreciated the fact that I didn't have to shop at the finest stores, but he pointed out that it wasn't wise to buy something we didn't need just because it was a bargain. "Do you really need ten photo albums for weddings we haven't even been invited to yet?" he asked.

It became increasingly embarrassing for him when we went out to dinner with friends from work and I pulled out a stack of coupons when the waiter brought the check, or the time our four-year-old daughter blurted out to a lady at church that "Mommy bought this dress for me at the Goodwill."

After John's income rose and I started bringing in extra money by working part-time for Bill, John felt it was time to buy new living room furniture. I disagreed. "Sure, our used furniture doesn't match and has a few stains from children and pets, but the same thing would happen to new furniture, so why waste the money? Besides, there's an estate sale coming up next weekend and we might find something there."

John nevertheless insisted that I budget for a new sofa and although I promised I would, I secretly continued to spend any extra money on "necessary" sale items.

My passion for bargain hunting turned into an obsession. I was addicted like a compulsive gambler, always thinking the next great treasure was just around the corner. I had passed up Saturday outings with the family because that was when the best garage sales occurred. John grew more and more frustrated with my addiction. He felt it was taking precious time away from the family and, anyway, was getting downright embarrassing.

The situation came to a head one night when we made a date; just the two of us would go out on a Saturday night and spend some much needed time without the little ones. I decided to leave the planning to John because if I made the plans, a coupon for dinner or dessert would surely be involved. John suggested we go to a movie that we both anxiously wanted to see. He said, "I'll call the babysitter so we can catch the seven o'clock show." My mind began to whirl and calculate: *The 7:00 P.M. show? What is he thinking? This is crazy. I can't go to a full-priced show.*

"John, honey," I said, "can't we go to the matinee instead? It's so much cheaper."

That was the straw that broke the camel's back. He looked me in the eye and said, "I can't believe you, Shelly. You've got five hundred dollars worth of candy hidden in a bureau drawer. You spend over two thousand dollars a year on gifts. But you won't pay three dollars extra to see a movie on a Saturday night. You complain about me never planning a date and when I do, you complain about that. We can afford the three dollars, I assure you."

The candy drawer and gift budget were an exaggeration, I rationalized to myself, and technically three dollars times two meant we would spend more like six dollars or even ten dollars more than a discounted matinee, especially if you counted the popcorn. I could see that I was carrying my thriftiness too far, but I couldn't stop myself. It was becoming a real obstacle in our marriage and family. I knew I had to change, but no amount of logic dispensed by my husband could stop me. I turned to my old friend Bill for help and inspiration. He has less expendable money than John and I, but he doesn't feel the need to shop "cheap." He lives from month to month and is content and comfortable with his simpler life.

A story Bill told me helped cure my compulsion to shop for bargains. While preparing a speech, I asked him what he remembered about his early childhood in San Francisco. I expected him to talk about persecution from other children or the physical pain associated with cerebral palsy. Wrong again, Shelly! Bill couldn't (or perhaps refused to) recall *any* painful memories. It was a happy, trouble-free time for him.

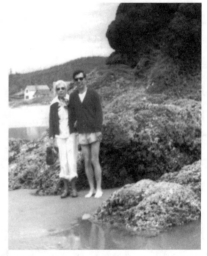

"I remember the teachers would take us out for sunbaths on the deck for a half-hour each day. The sun felt great on my skin. The teachers would tell us to roll over after fifteen minutes were up. I remember one evening my mom told me it was time to take a bath. I told her I didn't need to because I had already taken a bath, a sunbath. She laughed, but made me take a real bath with soap and water!"

I looked at Bill while he talked and I could see in his eyes how he truly cherished his joyous childhood. It brought tears of joy to my eyes. He is blessed with the ability to dwell on the positive and thinks of obstacles as exciting challenges.

I drifted off to my own childhood while he continued talking. I imagined myself on the beaches of Kauai with the surf up to my knees, waving back to my family on the beach. It was a beautiful, oft-repeated scene in my childhood. The sun and water felt so good. I knew without a doubt that my parents loved me and I loved them. It suddenly struck me how lucky I was to have grown up in a family that loved each other, no matter how much money was or was not in the bank. I also realized that, like Bill, I had no real obstacles; I wasn't handicapped because my family didn't have a lot of money. Rather, I was blessed because they loved me, just as my present family loves me and I love them. I finally saw clearly that I had allowed money — or the lack of it — to become an obstacle, an obsession, instead of a challenge. I didn't have to go overboard to save money and hoard bargain items. I had something you can't buy with money — love.

It has taken years, but with Bill as an example, I have changed my attitude towards money. Today, the last thing on my list of things I want to do is shop! (Besides, we could probably live for years off of the stuff I have in storage.) Now and then, I take a deep breath and treat the entire family to a full priced movie. Saturdays are now reserved for creating happy family memories. On hot summer days, we've

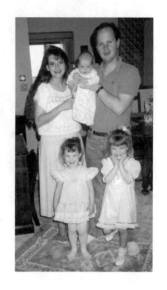

been known to go to the beach, play in the surf, and sunbathe. From Bill, I learned that I really don't have obstacles left over from my childhood, only challenges that require perseverance and time to overcome. Thank you, Bill Porter.

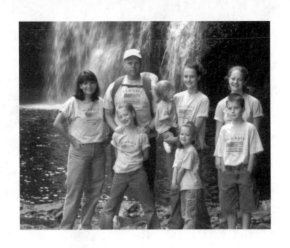

Chapter 10

Live Your Values

Bill is often asked, "What makes you tick? What makes you get up day after day, don a business suit, and sell door-to-door when you could stay home and collect disability payments?"

He answers, "I knew there was something I could do. I felt it deep inside. My mother told me I could do anything I set out to do and I believed her. I set out to work and nothing could make me take my eyes off that goal. When I was let go from the jobs the unemployment office set me up with, I was frustrated and discouraged, but I wouldn't let those feelings fester. I pushed them aside and kept going back. Eventually, I knew the right job would come my way. You must have faith in yourself and work hard. I learned that from my mother, my father, and God."

I marvel at the inner strength Bill Porter mustered during the 1980s when he cared for his ill mother and continued to work each day. "I had to go to work. I had to pay the bills," he'll tell you. Bill's admirable character traits are built upon a deep, internal value system.

Shortly before his mother passed away, I was asked to volunteer time for a youth group at my church. The goal of the group was to introduce young women to values they could use today and carry with them their entire life. Those values were: faith, divine nature, individual worth, knowledge, choice and accountability, good works, and integrity.

We had the girls choose someone they knew personally who exemplified the seven values and discuss how they were manifested. Well-respected parents, teachers, grand-parents, and friends were commonly cited as examples. To the surprise of the girls, I chose Bill Porter because more than anyone I know, he dramatically demonstrates the belief and practice of these seven values. In fact, he has believed and practiced them since childhood, when his parents taught him the importance of possessing the kind of internal values that one can rely on every day all through life. Bill's value system allowed him to function successfully in the face of major obstacles.

When it was my turn to discuss why I chose Bill as my example, I went down the list of values and talked about Bill's relationship with each one.

Faith

Irene Porter was a deeply religious woman. She taught her son to love God's wisdom in very practical terms, not abstractly, but by action, by the way one deals with all aspects of life, positive or negative. Irene didn't take the good things in life for granted; she gave thanks for every good turn of events, and she didn't see misfortunes as unlucky, insurmountable coincidences. Pouting or bemoaning one's downcast state were not options.

The Porter family attended church every Sunday where they prayed and gave thanks to a loving Heavenly Father who blessed their lives. Irene had faith that God didn't make mistakes; Bill's cerebral palsy was a part of Bill and thus a gift from the heavens above. In her heart, she believed God loved the Porter family and watched over them at every juncture. Irene taught Bill that faith carries one through the toughest of times. Bill learned that faith in God is synonymous with faith in humankind, which allowed him to see his customers as brothers and sisters.

Divine Nature

Irene and Ernest never doubted that Bill was a child of God who inherited divine qualities and gifts. He was taught that he had an obligation to discover and share these gifts. Irene taught him to be patient; it takes time to discover all God has given us. 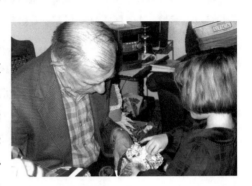 After many years of searching, Bill found he had a gift for selling, for gaining the trust of others because he earned it. Along his route, his friends and customers received more than products and smiles; they received from Bill an ability to recognize their own divine gifts and qualities.

Individual Worth

Irene felt it was a shame that parents of disabled children didn't recognize that a handicap can be a blessing in disguise. She understood the feelings of despair and sorrow, as she was initially devastated to learn her baby had cerebral palsy. But she quickly realized that Bill was special, that he was born into this world to teach important lessons to others. She believed her son was infinitely worthy of living in society, not in a hospital where his purpose on earth would be squelched. Consequently, Bill never developed an inferiority complex or a feeling of being handicapped. His mission was to be the best he could be, thereby inspiring others to learn by example that anything is possible.

Knowledge

Bill learned from his parents that knowledge is the key to a successful life. When Bill was diagnosed with cerebral palsy, Ernest and Irene educated themselves about the disease. Ernest quit his job as a salesman and found employment with a school for handicapped children, while Irene spent countless hours volunteering for United Cerebral Palsy. The Porters fought the establishment for years to get Bill into public schools. They knew that Bill needed a good education if he was ever going to make it on his own.

When Bill finally found work with Watkins, Incorporated, he learned everything he could about the company and their products. From his parents, Bill knew that one must thoroughly acquaint oneself about a subject before taking an action, such as selling door-to-door. Once a door is opened, Bill feels it's his duty to answer any questions about any products in his catalog. He educated himself about the industry as a whole and consistently bests the competition. He perfected the art of selling his products with a "money-back guarantee," which enlarged his client list and eventually made him the top sales producer in the Pacific Northwest.

He memorized the shopping habits and the likes and dislikes of more than five hundred clients. He is able to recite the names of clients who use vanilla when they bake and which ones insist on biodegradable soaps. Knowledge is power to Bill, and he never stops learning.

Choice and Accountability

Bill Porter certainly didn't choose to be born with cerebral palsy, but he and his parents had a choice of how to respond to the hand they'd been dealt. Many doctors and well-meaning friends suggested institutionalizing Bill. They told the Porters that there were many risks in keeping Bill at home. Instead, Irene and Ernest chose to love, nurture, and raise their child at home in spite of guaranteed hardships and sacrifices. They knew their medical bills would skyrocket and society wouldn't look kindly upon a family with a disabled child at home. Such children were to be hidden away in sanitariums and hospitals. But the choice to keep Bill was made without hesitation or regret.

Bill learned early on that choices exist; choices give one character and personality and distinguish good from evil. The knowledge that he had options was especially valuable to Bill when he first searched for employment.

"You have a choice, Bill," Irene told him. "You can get up and march right back down to that unemployment office and show them you're determined or stay home and stew." In theory it sounds simple, but many of us don't exercise our right to choose. Yet not making the right choice can lead to dead-end jobs and unfulfilled lives.

The knowledge that he had the power to pick and choose empowered Bill. When he deliberately chooses to ring a doorbell, he is formidable. One customer relates that when she saw Bill approach her house, she actually hid on the back porch and didn't answer the door. Bill knew she was at home and proceeded to knock on her back door. "I know you're home," he shouted. Out of complete embarrassment, the lady came out of hiding and bought a slew of products. Her husband read her the riot act when he came home.

"Why on God's earth did you buy from him when I told you not to?" he complained.

In her defense, she replied, "He's so upbeat and determined it's impossible to say no to him."

When the husband called to cancel the order, Bill guaranteed his money back in full if he wasn't satisfied. They are now long-time customers who welcome him into their home with open arms — and checkbooks.

Good Works

"Let your light so shine before men, that they may see your good works, and glorify your Father which is in heaven" (Matthew 5:16). Bill truly is a shining light in a dark world. He has spent his whole life working hard, struggling to learn everything he needed to become and stay independent. He is very much aware of and thankful for all the people who have come into his life to help him out. True, many of them receive a paycheck from Bill (remember, he is fiercely independent). He has accepted a few kind acts without payment: dinners from the ladies at church after his car accident, discounts on home improvements, new carpeting, and a sprinkler system, to mention a few.

Over the years, I have seen Bill watch for opportunities to "pay it forward." When a young teen who worked at a Wendy's Bill frequented was hit by a car, Bill was so concerned about her recovery he sent her flowers and chocolates and made numerous phone calls. On our business trips around the country, Bill always remembered to bring home thoughtful gifts for friends. He bought sweet smelling soaps and lotions for his physical therapist and souvenirs for his neighbors. I've seen him purchase candy from the kids selling door-to-door and then turn right around and give it back to them for resale or to eat themselves. Bill just shrugs his shoulders and says that chocolate gives him migraines anyway.

Integrity

When Bill sells a product to a client, there is never a hint of deception; he simply isn't capable of taking advantage of another human being. If you order a product from Bill, then you receive exactly what he promised, guaranteed by Bill and Watkins. To some business people, this righteous attitude may seem naive or unrealistic but it works; just look at his sales figures. When Bill reviews invoices in the evening, he sincerely looks out for his customers' interest. (Don't get me wrong; Bill loves the bottom line, too.) Every invoice is scanned to ensure that the numbers match up with the products.

In addition to delivering products for Bill, I was assigned the task of refunding

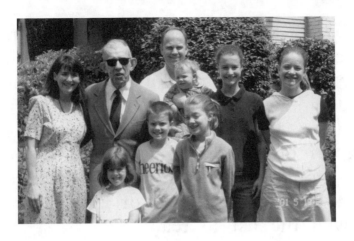

overpayments of even a few cents. In Bill's mind, two cents is no different from two hundred dollars; it's a matter of principle. Integrity takes precedence over money at all times. Integrity is the sphere that all of his business transactions revolve around. According to Bill, messing with honesty and integrity would cause widespread doom and gloom.

Brady Family Values

Bill's values are directly attributable to Irene's patient teachings, and I could just as well have chosen her as my example of a person who exemplifies the seven values we wished to impart upon the young girls at our church. She reminds me of how profoundly important it is for parents to teach their children well and to give them a value system they can believe in and carry with them through good times — and bad. My husband

and I try to teach these same values to our children. One evening many years ago, my family sat down at the kitchen table and discussed at length what our family mission should be. Knowing we couldn't include all the goals our large family hoped to accomplish, thoughts were openly shared and discussed and accepted or rejected. We narrowed the list to read:

Brady Family Mission

1. Be together forever.
2. Daddy and Mommy will watch over the children.
3. We will always be able to depend on each other in times of need.
4. We will always take the time to listen to each other.

We wrote the mission statement on a large piece of construction paper and hung it on our refrigerator. Ten years and four children later, this worn poster remains there today. Over the years as new goals were set — *Be kind, serve others, be thankful, love our neighbors, be honest* — we printed them on paper and taped them to the walls of the kitchen.

Although Bill and I belong to different faiths, we both believe in a higher power, one that includes us all as members of a large extended family, a family that loves and teaches each other. A verse I recently read encapsulates Bill Porter's life for me:

". . . and let us run with patience the race that is set before us, looking unto Jesus the author and finisher of our faith" (Hebrews 12:1,2).

That is how I see Bill Porter — patiently running a race, a race he is winning because of values his parents and God taught him. May the race continue to be long and fruitful for Bill, for I believe he is a true hero in the eyes of humanity and God.

Letters

Things You've Given Bill Porter

Through more than four decades, Bill trudged the streets and hills of Portland, Oregon, slightly bent, right arm pulled close in, left hand clutching his briefcase, walking, knocking on doors. He was an anonymous figure, known only to those on his sales route and perhaps to curious visitors to the neighborhood.

An article written by Tom Hallman, Jr., for the Portland *Oregonian* on November 27, 1995, introduced Bill Porter to a wider world and inspired articles in *Reader's Digest* and *Positive Living Magazine*. Television came next, with features on Bill appearing on *CBS This Morning* and eventually ABC's *20/20*. Millions of viewers watched and wept, and Bill's segment got the largest viewer response in the history of *20/20*.

The response has touched Bill deeply. As the letters poured in, he began to see a glimpse of an additional purpose to his life. Bill and I would sit together in his living room reading every single letter. Tears came to our eyes as we read the heart-felt outpourings of pain and joy from our new friends.

Bill commented how these letters gave him so much hope and strength. It was like a circle of love and inspiration, confirming that what you give away comes back tenfold.

Choosing which letters to include here was one of the most difficult tasks we faced in putting this book together. Thank you to all who wrote, and know that each and every letter is precious to Bill and to me.

December 1, 1998

Dear Mr. Porter,

I believe this is the first time in my 44 years that I have been moved to respond to a TV show. After seeing your story on 20/20 last week, I simply had to write to let you know how inspirational you are. I don't think anyone could have watched and learned about you without feeling moved. You are an uncommon and exceptional human being, though I'm certain that your modesty prevents you from even acknowledging that you are special in any way. This is just another facet of you that makes you so remarkable.

How lucky you were to have a mother who could instill such quiet confidence in you, and how lucky she, to have such a caring and hardworking son to look after her in her later years. You can be sure that before her cruel disease robbed her of her personality, she was indeed proud of you and grateful for all of your efforts on her behalf. Who wouldn't be proud to have such a son. You both completed each other's lives.

This world is in desperate need of positive role models and heroes, and while I'm sure you are uncomfortable with this praise and feel it is unwarranted, you are indeed someone that all of us can look up to. Your work ethic and determined spirit is the "right stuff" of which we see so little these days.

Thank you for renewing my faith in mankind you are wonderful!

I wish you good health, continued success in your business endeavors and most of all, happiness you have earned it and certainly deserve it!

Abby
Scarborough, Ontario

Mr. Porter,

I would just like to say that in a world where so many look for the smallest reasons to give up you are an inspiration. Not for what you have overcome but for showing the rare traits of determination and personal pride. I admire you, not for the adversities you have overcome but for your GOOD SOUL. The world needs more people like you.

Thomas W. Newton
New Carlisle, Ohio

April 12, 1998

Dear Mr. Porter,

My name is Pam Noblet, and I'm 17 years old. A couple of months ago I saw a 20/20 special about you. Right away I felt proud to know that TV has something positive on it. I wanted to find out how to write to you, so I wrote on the computer to 20/20. They replied and gave me your address. The reason why I'm writing is to tell you that you remind me a lot of my friend Matt.

Matt also has Cerebral Palsy, but he's in a wheelchair. Matt has enough strength to lead an entire football team. I met Matt about three years ago through a mutual friend. To tell you the truth, the first thing I noticed about Matt is not the wheelchair but his great big smile. Over the years that I've known him I've become really fond and protective of him. Matt and I have a lot of fun together. We go shopping, to the movies, baseball games, and do what ever else I want to do. People tell me that it takes a special person to be friends with someone like Matt.

Well I'll tell you something, I don't think I'm a special person. I think Matt is one of the easiest people to be friends with. His fun, outgoing personality makes me want to reach over and hug him.

I just wanted you to know I think you're a great man. You give a lot of encouragement to all people. Thanks for sharing your story with 20/20 so that many people can be educated. Thanks again.

Your New Friend,
Pam Noblet
Bozrah, Connecticut

Dear Mr. Bill,

I just saw your story on 20/20. I must tell you that you have given me an inspiration like I have never experienced before. I am 34 years old, and I have been putting myself through college in hopes to get into medical school. I work full time and find it very hard sometimes to complete the complex course work needed to enter medical school. For the past few weeks, I have been thinking about giving up on my dream. Although I have gotten my degree, I still needed to complete a few extra, very difficult classes to prepare myself. With work and lack of money to pay for such classes, I began to get discouraged.

But when I saw your story, I realized my problems are minor and my heart was filled with a joy I have never encountered before. I had tears in my eyes when I heard you were struck by a car. I thought I was about to hear you were killed. The world would be a much better place with a lot more Bill Porters. You have given me the inspiration needed to carry on. I feel as though I have been touched by an Angel and my heart has been lifted. I hope you are doing well this Christmas. I truly thank you from the bottom of my heart for what you have given me.

Merry Christmas

Michael
Baton Rouge, Louisiana

Dear Bill,

I saw you in Winston at the Amway seminar and you were the singular best speaker I have ever heard. You will always remain with me. My grandchild will know you and admire you. You are a blessing from God. All men I have ever known pale in your light. I have always said that your actions are so loud I can't hear what you are saying. You need no microphone, I can hear you every day of my life. As a salesperson, I have been able to overcome a grossly overblown ego with just a glance at your picture. I have been permanently cured of excusitis. How can I best serve you now?

Brian Ethridge
Denver, North Carolina

Dear Mr. Porter,

My name is Milton. I am a petty officer in the U.S. Navy. I am currently stationed at naval station Roosevelt Roads, Puerto Rico.

I am writing you in order to express my admiration for you. I have been asked my whole life who my hero was; who I looked up to. I could never give an answer. I never had anyone that lived up to my expectations of a hero. Now, if anyone asks me who my hero is, I can tell them with pride and certainty, "Mr. Bill Porter of Oregon is my hero."

Thank you, Mr. Porter, for giving me a hero.

Sincerely,
Milton
Ceiba, Puerto Rico

Bill and Shelly,

I heard Bill speak at the Home Base conference in Colorado Springs. My name is Frank Toms, and I am the Marketing Director for Aqua Mix Inc., one of the Home Base's suppliers. I am 32 years old, and I guess you can say I am part of the "me" generation.

It is not often that an individual has changed my attitude/outlook about my life. Bill has shown me the true meaning of spirit, determination, and pride.

Bill, I understand you don't want anyone to feel sorry for you. Based on the accomplishments you have made in your life, I do not pity you. However, please understand that you make perfectly healthy people like myself feel truly blessed for the gifts we were given. I no longer take a lot of things for granted, which in turn has made me a wiser better person. I cannot thank you enough for that wonderful gift.

So, to both of you and your families, I wish you a Merry Christmas.

Frank Toms
Huntington Beach, California

Dear Bill:

I saw you last night for the first time on 20/20. It was a rerun of their original segment on "The Oregonian" story.

It was truly inspirational, Bill. I too am in sales, and know full well how depressing and discouraging this field can be. You however seem to have transcended everything that can discourage a sales representative.

In the first few minutes of the airing, I thought to myself "how much of a disadvantage you must be operating." You see I was thinking of the computer age, the Internet, facsimile technology, etc., not your "so-called" disability.

But as your story continued to unfold, I soon realized that I was missing the point. So often we forget that we are human, we need human touch, feeling, conversation, companionship, to help one another. Whether it be to ask for assistance or — harder yet — allowing ourselves to be helped by others that observe our need and show a willingness to help us.

I guess if there is one thing I appreciate the most about your story it's your total humility. I was touched by you and your life story.

Best wishes to you Bill.

Sincerely,
Barry

P.S. Shelly Brady, you are a very special person, may God continue to bless you.

Dear Bill Porter,

It's Christmas day. Last night I saw your story on 20/20. I was very touched by the kind of person you are, Bill Porter.

In my life I strive every day to think about what I can do to become more influential and have a greater impact on those around me. I think on grand scales — world famous, etc. I think to myself "What can I do in life to become more recognizable and be able to reach more people?" Last night your story gave me the answer. Although not the answer I was necessarily searching for — but an answer nonetheless.

The answer was nothing. I should do nothing but that which I am supposed to do on a daily basis. He who would be King must be servant of all. In my haste to reach some sort of throne in the world, I have forgotten what it is to be lost among the masses doing what I need to do and not worry about who sees me or what consequences may or may not arise because of it.

You are an inspiration — you are a godly man — and you are a King among men.

Then again, you've earned it. God will crown you for the life you have led — your mother, I know, is VERY proud of you.

I hope one day I might meet the man they call Bill Porter.

Aaron Hutchins
Patchogue, New York

Hi!

I saw your story on 20/20 and was moved to loving tears. For me, your story increased my faith in people, especially now when there are so many bad things occurring daily. It must have been meant for me to watch your story because I was just channel flipping. I caught the beginning of the story which I thought was simply about a door-to-door salesman, which just wasn't interesting. But something (that little voice that we should listen to more often) told me to watch it.

Your story also increased my faith, because my life has been horrible because of the sickening wrong doings of others, including parents, family, and people I thought were friends. Daily, I wished I wasn't here, but to see you, Bill, go through every day without complaining taught me a lesson and reminded me of the never ending faith and determination my grandparents had — something I could never understand until now. Thanks for being human — something that the majority of us forget that we are!

Take care and God bless!

Tamra Marie Burgess
Edgewater, New Jersey

And God bless Shelly Brady and her family.

13 Jan, 00

Dear Bill,

Just a note to say hello. Got a nice update from Mrs. Brady. Sorry you haven't been up to par and hope things have improved.

I'm a 63-year-old navy retiree. I've been around a lot of guys in the submarine service and in Vietnam. I've got to say that of all the great veterans and servicemen I've known, that you are on the top of my list for guts and peserverence. I truly admire you and the way you have conducted your life.

I'm certain that some day, far in the future I hope, you will stand before your God, and he will tell you that you are one of his proudest creations. When that time comes, I'm sure your reward will be great.

I wish you the very best, now, and in the days to come. I think you should lighten up some and take it easy. Enjoy the fruits of your excellent labor.

Best wishes.

Lloyd Alfred, USN(SS), Retired
McDonald, Pennsylvania

Mr. Porter,

I first saw your story on 20/20 last year and recorded it based on the promo that they did prior to the show. It brought tears to my eyes. Rarely have I seen that type of media do such a touching and inspiring piece. I suffer from cluster migraine headaches that have ruined my life for 18 years. I no longer feel sorry for myself. Instead, I am ashamed at how much I have blamed my headaches for limiting my options in life. You are a true inspiration, Bill, and I hope someday to shake your hand. I wish you all the best, and a very Merry Christmas (tomorrow). Please take care of yourself, and if you are ever in the area, please let me know via e-mail so I can get that chance to shake your hand . . . and perhaps give you a hug.

If Watkin's could bottle the determination and huge heart you have, I would like very much to purchase some! God bless you, and God bless Shelly for being there for you.

All the best to you.

Max Kane
Gladwin, Michigan

Dear Shelly,

I realize that you are being bombarded with mail. However, I just had to write. I was not there the weekend you and Mr. Porter spoke, but I did see the segment on the news program and heard about you the following weekend at the Convention in Richmond, Virginia.

Mr. Porter is amazing. There have been a couple of people throughout my life with speech impediments. My grandmother was deaf, but still talked in a slurred pattern. God works in amazing ways. Growing up with this helped me understand two different people in college. One was an African from Kenya and had a thick accent. I was able to understand him the first time, so we traded. I helped him with studies and he taught me his language. There was also another person who had CP or MS, and he was easy for me to understand. Also, in my workplace there are people with speech difficulties and it is wonderful to be able to help them when others don't or won't take the time to help.

You are also amazing. With raising a family and still taking time to help this gentleman makes you an Angel in my eyes. When I saw the story a poem that I keep at my desk to remind me daily about a smile and kindness came to mind. I thought I would share it with you.

My life shall touch a dozen lives before
   this day is done,
Leave countless marks for good or ill
   ere sets the evening sun,
This is the wish I always wish, the
   prayer I always pray;
Lord, may my life help others lives it
   touches by the way.

You and Bill have certainly touched a lot of lives through the Britt Spring Leaderships.

Thank you for letting me share with you and may God be with you and your family.

With Love, Debbie

It is Christmas Eve, and I just finished watching the segment that 20/20 did on your story. I must say that I feel blessed to have turned on the television at the exact time that I did. I am 27, and recently relocated to Ohio from Missouri for my husband's job.

My husband is scheduled to go out on the road tomorrow morning at 6:30. He was also working at Thanksgiving, so this will be the second holiday I have spent alone. I must admit that I was feeling very sorry for myself until now. I was both inspired and motivated by your story. I once read that the quality of one's life is not measured by the things one acquires, but by the lives one touches. If this is true (and I am sure it is), then the quality of your life must be immeasurable. I would be willing to bet that your story alone has shaped more lives than you could ever imagine. I am so thankful that you shared your life with others. I will be sure to "count my blessings" more often. Thank you, and have a wonderful Christmas and a SAFE New Year!

Dawn LaRocco
Westerville, Ohio

January 3, 2000

Dear Mr. Porter,

My name is Troy Nelson. I am originally from South Dakota where I was adopted as a baby and raised. I am now 23 years old and have been spending half of my life trying to make a living writing songs. The past few years I have suffered from depression and anxiety which has greatly affected my career choice as a musician. I have been down on myself about my songs and my ability to write them. I always think that I have only a certain time limit before I am too old to be accepted or taken seriously.

After learning about your story of persistence and determination, it has taught me to do what I do and to do it the best that I can do, no matter what people say and that there is no time limit on life when you have a drive that will last forever. After hearing your story, I prayed to God that there is someone like you, an example for all humans. Even though you hear it everyday, and will continue to hear it in the future, THANK YOU.

Sincerely,

Troy M. Nelson
Seattle, Washington

P.S. I am writing a song about your journey and how it's helped me. I would love for you to hear it, and if you do, let me know how I can get it to you. I would be deeply honored.

Wednesday December, 1999

Dear Shelly,

I can't begin to tell you how thankful I am that Bill Porter has an assistant like you. I talked to you on the telephone yesterday for the first time. You are obviously a caring, warm-hearted individual. You have sacrificed in order to help a man who, because of limitations beyond his control, has not had an easy time providing for himself. I can't tell you how much I appreciate that.

I remember Bill Porter. I grew up on Hewett Boulevard in the southwest hills of Portland. Often times, I saw Bill Porter walking from one home to another, not fully aware of his purpose. I certainly was not aware of his history or the daily struggles and challenges he was facing. I have many regrets about not being more perceptive of this man, who is now a daily inspiration both personally and professionally.

I am now 34 years old, married to a wonderful woman, and father of three boys (most recently twin boys who arrived four weeks ago). Like Bill, I am also in sales and have been for the past nine years. Bill Porter has inspired me to be a more thoughtful, self-motivated, and caring individual. My

185

wife, Ingrid, has read the articles about Bill. Together we have watched the program on 20/20. We even ordered a copy of the tape to share with family and friends who missed the program. I can assure you that when my boys are older, they too will know of Bill Porter.

I have saved copies of all the articles I could find regarding Bill. I have shared his story with all the salespeople that now report to me, as well as our customer service group and management. I took a Dale Carnegie sales course two years ago and shared his story with everyone in the class. His story is a humbling one, and, as you can imagine, put most of the class into tears, which is often times the case when his story is told.

I apologize for the length of the message, but I just wanted you to know how much both of you are appreciated and that you have touched the lives of many. Please take this check and buy something that can be donated to a local charity (i.e., Morrison Center, homeless shelter, women's shelter, etc.). I trust your judgment.

I hope some day to meet Mr. Porter and thank him personally for the positive impact he has had on my life. Until then, please pass along my thanks and best wishes.

Happy Holidays!

Rob Williams
Kent, Washington

Dear Mr. Porter,

I truly enjoyed your recent interview on 20/20. Your story left me so inspired to work hard and NOT complain so much! The next day I told my ten-year-old son about you and he, too, was moved by your story.

Needless to say, my son has been more co-operative with his chores, less procrastinating, and much more attentive. I attribute his new-found maturity much in part to your story and the fine example you are.

Today, my son announced that you were his hero. I wanted you to know.

Most Sincerely,

Hillary Roberts
Keyport, New Jersey

(To learn more about Hillary's nonprofit organization inspired by Bill's story go to www.blankiedepo.org.)

Just wanted to drop by and congratulate you on persevering in a world that is difficult enough for us whose greatest disability is our own attitudes. Saw the segment on 20/20 tonight (Dec. 24) and can only hope to achieve some minute measure of success that you have been able to. You are truly an inspiration to those of us that feel like there is no tomorrow for us in the "selling game." I will face a new year with a different attitude because of you.

Thanks Bill,
John K. Wadsworth
Stockton, California

Dear Bill,

I listened to your story Christmas Eve night on the 20/20 show and had to write you a letter and tell you that your story was an inspiration to me. I work as a police officer in a small town in southern Minnesota, and my wife is a nurse at the state hospital in Fergus Falls, Minnesota. So we both had to go to work Christmas Eve and that's when I had the opportunity to hear about you. I also work at the local high school about two to three days a week and work with kids that are in gangs or come from broken homes or homes without love. I didn't know your mom, Bill, but she was one of those people with an unconditional love. I learned that from hearing your story. I don't think I would have heard about you turning out to be a good person if your mom hadn't been a good person also. I wish these kids I work with had a Mrs. Porter or a Bill Porter in their lives and the world would be a better place.

Bill, if you ever get to Minnesota I am inviting you to the school where I work to share you with the students. I learned once that the meaning of success is getting up one more time after you fall down — BUT now I have a new definition!!!! BILL PORTER!

Well maybe some day I can meet you and sit down and visit with you if you have time. I wish we were closer. Oh by the way, my family also used and sold, for goodness sakes, Watkins Products, and I even think they're from Winona, Minnesota.

Friends Officer,
Jimmy Hansen

Stewart Police Department
Stewart, Minnesota

Dear Bill,
I'm 17 years old and before I went to bed

the other night I saw your story on TV. It made me cry very hard. I really admire you for what you have done throughout your life and that you have stuck to it without giving up. I one day hope to have as much determination as you do. It just made me think of what I am going to do with my life and if I'll ever be as determined and happy about what I'm doing as you are. Your story just really made me think a lot. Thank you for sharing it with us!

Missy
Youngsville, North Carolina

12/31/99
Shelly and Bill,

We hope that the New Year brings you health and happiness! I can't help but to say that when I think of you or tell someone your story, Bill, I always seem to say that "I love you" because of who you are! If only I could be half of the person you are! You have touched so many. And Shelly I am very grateful to you that Bill and your lives crossed paths. To know that you have been a longtime friend to him is comforting! He has brought a universal message that the heart is the power of all and that what we "see" is only part of what we get!

Thanks for keeping us posted!

> Rhonda & Steve Stenersen
> Post Falls, Idaho

Dear Mr. Porter,

Our class viewed your story on 20/20, and was very inspired by your sense of dedication and willingness to press on in life despite the difficulty of the circumstances. Your humble and gentle spirit especially influenced the children, as their letters clearly indicate. You are a person greatly to be admired, and have made a positive and lasting impact on all of the students who have learned of you. I have no doubt that God Himself is greatly appreciative of the many things you have done to make the world a better place. We hope the best of everything for you, as you continue on in your work. You are a blessing to everyone who has come into contact with you.

> With great respect and admiration,

> Keith
> Green Elementary, fifth grade teacher

December 20, 1997

Dear Mr. Bill Porter,

I was watching the ABC News Program 20/20. I was touched very much by the story about you. You see my wife and I are mentally handicapped. Both myself, Greg, and my wife, Val, can walk and talk, but we don't drive due to our motor coordination, etc. You, Mr. Porter, have more of a disability than me or my wife. I am not mad at you. What I am just trying to say, both my wife and I are adults with learning disabilities. You have had a hard time in your life, and the story about you brought tears to our eyes. You gave us hope and courage that the world of the disabled can live a normal life, not locked away in an institution, but in the community of the non-disabled.

I have a neck-shoulder injury, the story about you gives me hope to cope with it.

You take care of yourself, I can't think of anything else to say.

> Happy Holidays and Thank you,
> Greg and Valerie A. Gibson
> Somerville, New Jersey

P.S. from my wife, Val: Thank you for making us realize what we have and how grateful we should be.

December 24, 1997
20/20 News Show
New York, New York

Dear Sir or Madam,

I am compelled to write to you after seeing your story on Bill Porter. He has changed my life. I no longer accept excuses for myself or for others at what they or I can't do, only what I and others can do. I am awe-inspired at what he does on a daily basis without a whine or a complaint. I don't think most people could do this in a lifetime.

His perseverance, determination, and true grit are something to be admired and if more people followed that the world would be a better place. When people talk about hero's, great athletes, movie stars, and politicians come to mind. They don't hold a candle to Bill Porter. For me there is no greater hero than Bill Porter. He is head and shoulders above the rest.

I salute Bill Porter for all that he stands for and I hope that America will take him into their arms and hearts and embrace him too.

I thank you for doing a story on a true hero. I hope you do a follow-up on him so we can all know how he is doing.

Sincerely,
Michelle Solon Rhome
Bardonia, New York

January 2, 1998

Dear Mr. Porter:
We are the family that called you last Sunday. We have two sons, Erik, who is almost 5, and a newborn, Mikal. We showed your story to Erik and he has asked us numerous times since if he could see "that nice man" again. He has asked how you are, and we, as a family, have been praying for you. Every one of us, of whom has been given this gift of life, has been given their own package. Each has special treasures that only that one person can give, and each has their limitations. As a mother, I realize what a gift your mother gave you. She believed in you.

Thank you for allowing 20/20 to share with us your life. It meant a lot to us. Your life is an encouragement to us, and your mothers' life encourages us to instill in our boys that whatever their gifts or talents may be, to put forth their best efforts, and do it with integrity, and to walk humbly before the Lord. In short, we hope to impart in our boys the same sense of determination, perseverance and self-worth that your mother imparted in you.

We pray for your speedy recovery and God's richest blessing on your life.

Sincerely yours, Greg and Angela Winters
Ridgecrest, California

Bill Porter,

I love you! You are my best friend. Thank you for letting us watch your story on T.V. I hope you feel well soon. I love you. God loves you Mr. Bill. I like very much how nice you are to everybody and I like your smile.

Love, Erik

Dear Bill Porter,

I watched the 20/20 that you were on, and I thought it was the best thing that I have ever seen before in my life. I think that you are so courageous. You have a lot of courage to ignore all of the other people and just go on with your dream. That is what I am going to do. I am not going to let anybody tell me that I can't do what my dream may be. I am so happy for you and the way that you are so nice to everybody. I think that whatever you want to do you may do it because you have the courage to do it. I think that that is so cool that you do what you do, I don't think that I could do what you do. All of the other companies that have not let you work for them, I think that they are just plain dumb. I bet that you would and could do much better than the other people selling stuff, way better. You are doing the best job that anybody could ever do. I think that you are doing a good job since you broke your hip. I hope you get better and I think that you should keep up the good work. You should be the leader in everybody's life. You are a great and fantastic role model. Keep up the good work.

From,

Lauren

Dear Bill Porter,

I watched 20/20 in reading class. My name is Erika, and I think you are the greatest nicest person I have ever seen before because you go around the whole town and go to door to door selling things and you are helping people out. I can't believe you can stand being called names or not being excepted at any business place. Even though people say things about you don't care you just keep going on and never stop. You taught kids a lesson and that is to never give up or stop thinking about your dream! And you have inspired me to go for my lifelong dream. You are my guide forever! You have done a good deed for everyone!!!

Sincerely,
Erika

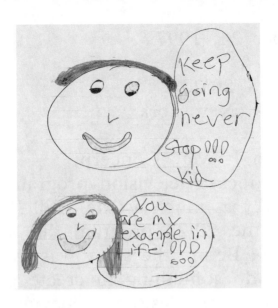

Dear Mr. Porter,

Hello my name is Rachel. You probably don't know me. The only reason I know you is because I just saw your story on 20/20. It made me cry. I am 10 years old. I can't believe you never give up. You should be happy for that. Because if I were you I'd give up. Also you don't take no for an answer. Now that is amazing. You know what if you still have trouble hearing you can buy hearing aids.

Yours truly,
Rachel

P.S. Call me

December 24, 1997

ABC-TV - 20/20
New York, New York

To Whom It May Concern:
Rarely does a television program move me emotionally as much as the "Bill Porter" segment of the 20/20 program did almost two weeks ago. Before the show was over, I knew I had to do something to create positive reinforcement of desired behavior. I wrote down the name of the segment and the employer of Mr. Porter as well as his hometown. With the Christmas season in full swing, I did not have the time to begin this letter and the others I will write until today.

I don't believe I have ever written to a television station to compliment them on their programming. This is primarily because I do not believe the majority of programming on any of the major networks is worthy of compliments. However, with the broadcast of the "Bill Porter" segment, it is apparent that there is still hope.

Bill Porter embodies all of the good qualities of human nature we all should strive to possess. He is an excellent example for anyone to follow. From an employers perspective, he is dependable, loyal, driven, motivated, confident, selfless, conscientious, talented, dedicated, and the list goes on and on. From a human perspective he embodies all of these same traits and is caring, concerned, loving, a friend to all, and a good citizen and neighbor. He is the man I hope to be and want my kids to grow up to be like. He is Bill Porter in spite all of his physical deviations from the norm. His heart is clearly visible through the way he lives his life. Bill Porter reminds me of my dad with his work ethic. He doesn't feel society owes him anything and he works hard for what he has.

While I watched this segment, my emotions welled up inside of me and escaped as tears of joy. I was so overwhelmed with how truly exceptional this man is without even considering his physical differences. We need for all stations to find the Bill Porter's of the world and feature their lives in segments or documentaries like yours. This is the programming we need for our fathers, mothers, and children to see and having seen, hopefully strive to develop the qualities Bill Porter has. Your station is to be commended on this quality piece of work and encouraged to replace the garbage that permeates all daily programming with human-interest stories like this. I cannot remember a program that has so stirred my inner being as much as this one. It motivated me to get off the couch and do something. I'm sure I am not alone in that regard.

I cannot say enough about the quality of

this piece. I want to personally thank those responsible for the Bill Porter piece for doing such an excellent job showcasing one of America's truly great resources, Bill Porter.

Thanks again and Happy Holidays!

> With best regards, I am Sincerely yours,
> William M. Magee
> Abita Springs, Louisiana

Cc: NBC-TV; CBS-TV; FOX-TV; The Watkins Company; Bill Porter; The Learning Channel; The Discovery Channel

January 19, 1998
Dear Mr. Porter,

I have been meaning to sit down to write you this letter since I first heard your story on 20/20 in December. I even looked up the program information on the 20/20 website pages and printed it out (with photos) as a reminder of a remarkably courageous person.

I would simply like to thank you for allowing your story to be told. I understand from the telecast that you were somewhat reluctant. Let me just say that your story, Mr. Porter, has changed the way I look at myself and for this I want to thank you.

I once read that courage is the most important virtue because without it you can't do anything else with consistency. You, Mr. Porter, are living proof and the embodiment of all, that I believe, "courage" means.

I too have been waging a war against the odds — for almost twelve years now I have been battling cancer. A mere drop in the bucket though, when compared to your sixty-five years. I am not, however, courageous like you. What an incredible gift you possess to have been such a fighter, such a doer, such an incredibly strong being, right from the beginning. I wasn't diagnosed with cancer until I was 37 years old. Up until that time I never really understood how precious this life is. Well, I almost lost sight of that until I was lucky enough to catch 20/20 that Friday night — when I saw you.

Your story has touched me in a way that I find hard to explain. I think you know what I mean though, Mr. Porter. Just the mere fact that the segment on you drew the largest response of any story in 20/20's history is a testament of how many lives you touched.

Again, thank you, Mr. Porter, for taking the time to share your life. You will always be an inspiration to me, especially at those times when I don't feel like fighting cancer anymore. Just thinking about you will set things right.

God's speed, Mr. Porter. Stay well. It's like

I keep telling my oncologist — it's so much more than medicine.

With deepest regards,

Maryann Wells
Streetsville, Ontario, Canada

December 14, 1997

Dear Bill,

Enjoyed seeing the piece on you on 20/20. My heart swelled with pride for the accomplishment in your life. The great satisfaction you must take in making your own way in the world.

My oldest brother is now 55 and suffered from an injury at birth. He still lives with our mother in Ohio. Mother is now 78. Sonny never developed the power of speech or fine motor skills, like buttoning buttons or zipping a zipper. He has spent his life in my parents home being loved and well cared for. The past 15 years he has been able to go to a sheltered workshop. The bus picks him up every morning and drops him off late in the afternoon. The thought of being self-sufficient, holding a job would have been but a dream, but he remains sweet and pleasant — just like you. Your goodness and kindness came shining through!!!

Through my brother I have a sincere sense of your accomplishments. How proud your mother would have been. My best wishes and good thoughts go out to you on this Christmas holiday.

I've included a small gift for under your tree.

Steve Graumlich
Savannah, Georgia

Dear Bill,

I was thrilled to see you on 20/20 on TV. It seems like just yesterday when we were going to Grout Center. I am certainly glad you were able to be a salesman as you always wanted to be. I am sorry to hear about your mother. As I remember her, she was a very wonderful lady, as were all our mothers. You remember I lost my mother shortly after I graduated from Grout. Those were hard days. As I remember you went to the Salvation Army Camp right after school was out in 1950. I don't remember if you were there in 1951 or not. That is the last time I had significant contact with any of the students that went to Grout Center. My dad remarried then in September of 1950. After I graduated from Grout, I was able to attend Franklin High School and graduate in 1954. I was able to graduate from Brigham Young University in chemistry and also graduate from the University of Utah Law School. I worked in the United States Patent Office as a Patent Examiner until 1990 when I had to retire on disability because my spinal cord was compromised, parazlying my arms. I have been living in Utah since 1990.

The Lord has blessed me with a family and a career. We are both so fortunate that we were able to accomplish something with our lives and fit into society. It must have been a struggle for you to keep up your sales route. It seems now that handicapped people have the attitude they want to be compensated for their handicap. I think both of us have struggled to give something to society and to do the best we can with our handicap. I have had a lot of help from people and I imagine you have too. I have not demanded help and it saddens me that some of the people in the handicapped movement demand accommodations that are unreasonable.

Have you kept track of any of the kids we knew? I have completely lost track of everyone. I have seen David Ingerson and Neil Firm in Portland three times in the past thirty years. As I remember it, they were on the staff of the CP Center in southeast Portland. I think the last time I had any contact was in 1979 or 1980. I heard Janie Poor and Morris Foss got married. Do you ever see them? My wife is typing this letter for me, and if it is too difficult for you to write to me, don't worry about it. If you are able to give me a call, we might be able to understand each other. I am out of practice, however, and the general public has trouble understanding me at times. My phone number is in the evening.

Delbert Phillips
Springville, Utah

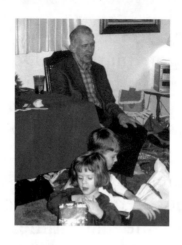

Afterword

by *Bill Porter*

To me, the thought that others will find my life worthy of an entire book is unbelievable. Even more unbelievable is this beautiful book that Shelly has written. When she asked me if I had anything to add to the book, my answer was "You bet. I want to thank all the people who have contributed to my life story."

So many people have helped me throughout my life and made my life better. I wish I could thank each and every one of them, but I can't. My gratitude to them is so great that it would take me years and years just to express it, so a simple thank you will have to suffice.

Many people have been generous with gifts,

such as Mark and Lizzette Rolls of Primerica Financial Services who gave us a trip to Disneyland. Others have given me the gift of time. Father Arthur Dernbach, the priest at Saint Thomas More Catholic Church in Portland, was always there to talk with me and advise me. The church secretaries and members were always kind and welcoming to me, too. I ate my lunch in the churchyard every day for years, and Father Dernbach would join me and we would sit and chat. Later, when Mother was ill and passed away, Father Dernbach performed the memorial funeral service and everyone in the congregation comforted me through my sorrow and loss.

Shelly deserves my thanks for all the help she has given me over the years, and especially for helping me tell my story. I appreciate the Brady family's generosity in sharing her with me and for being my "family," too. Thanks to all the people who saw my story in the newspaper or on television and sent me letters. My biggest thank you, though, goes to my customers whose orders, small and large, made my life possible.

I never thought my life had meaning, and I didn't live it as though it was important to anyone except those close to me. My message to everyone who reads this book is that your life is important, too. Think about each person you meet each day of your life and what effect you might have upon them, for good or ill. It isn't always the big decisions that make a difference in our lives; more often, it's the little ones. The extra smile or wave; calling a friend who is ill; going out of your way to help someone whether they ask or not. Each of you has the same opportunity to inspire others as I do, simply by living your life as best you can. People tell me that I have touched thousands of lives, but what I think is that hundreds and thousands of people have helped me. Thank you, each of you, and every time you ask yourself if you can make a difference, remember this answer: You bet you can.

List of Illustrations

211

Acknowledgments

There are so many people I wish to express my appreciation to, so many who have taught me great lessons in teamwork, friendship, and support. My greatest fear is that I will miss someone. If I do I hope that they will forgive me and know they are in my heart.

My greatest blessing, love, and joy come from my family. I am so thankful for a patient, loving husband. John has supported me all the years as I have delivered Watkins products, shopped, and cleaned for Bill (even when we had no clean clothing or milk in our own fridge). He's lovingly cared for our children while I flew around the country inspiring others with Bill's story. He's kindly picked up countless pizzas on his way home from work when time and again I didn't get around to fixing dinner while working on this book. He's helped me figure out how to balance my role as a homemaker with my speaking career. He's also encouraged and helped me with ideas for this book. He is my best friend.

My children mean the world to me: Michelle, Katrina, Teressa, Kevin, Erica, and

Emily. I appreciate their continuous support and patience with me. (One daughter has informed me that when she grows up, she wants to be a mom, but she won't write a book. She'll just play with her children.) They cooked, cleaned, played with the ones briefly missing mommy, and changed the baby's diapers when I was out of town or locked away in my room writing. They love me unconditionally. For the past several years, they, along with their father, helped deliver Bill's products. They help me clean Bill's house. They bring me great joy. They are my greatest moments!

I love and appreciate my mother, Harriette Hankel, so much. She is the busiest person I know but always takes the time to listen to me. She has spent hours reading every chapter over and over, offering her suggestions.

To all my parents — Gary (Dad), Linda, John, and Harriette (Mom) — thanks for helping me grow up.

To my sisters and brothers — Ann, Shayne, Chris, Che, Israel, Glenn, and Jennifer — thank you for always being there. To Che for making me promise if I ever wrote this book that some of the proceeds should be earmarked to help someone else, resulting in New World Library's contribution to United Cerebral Palsy.

I could not have written this book or trav-

eled with Bill without the help of my "team."
To my in-laws, Elwood and Melba Brady,
thank you for lovingly tending your grandchildren — my babies — so many times over
the past few years. It's comforting to know
my children are in the best of hands when I
am gone or busy at the computer.

Thanks also to Diane Young and Sheila
Painter, friends as close as family, who also
spent countless hours tending my little ones
so I could travel or work on this book.

I mention with gratitude the many friends
who helped me with the book by reading,
proofing, and sharing their thoughts and
ideas with me: Wendi Stephens, Tesa
Stephens, Polly Johnson, Rhonda Carter, and
Tricia Craft. Thank you so much for your
help and thank you most of all for your
friendship.

I would like to thank everyone at Nation-
wide Speakers Bureau, especially our agent,
Dan Savage, for representing Bill and me
these past few years and opening doors for
us to speak all over this great country to
people from all over this great world.

To our good friend Robert J. King, who
got the ball rolling for the most amazing
movie project ever! To Carey Nelson-Burch
who hooked Rob up with Dan Angel, Billy
Brown, and Forest Whitaker who helped roll
that ball faster and faster. To everyone at
TNT, including producers David A. Rose-

mont and Warren Carr, who made it happen. To Steven Schachter who helped write the screenplay and directed the movie *Door to Door*. To the actors and crew on the set of the movie who poured their hearts into their work. And last but not least, to William H. (Bill) Macy who co-wrote and starred as my friend Bill Porter in the movie. To all of these wonderful people, thanks for seeing Bill's story as the wonderful piece of life that it is and for making a movie that will touch millions. And thanks, Bill Macy, for writing the foreword to this book, for sitting in a make-up chair for hours each day, for capturing the spirit and heart of Bill Porter as you played him, and for being our friend.

I would like to thank Katie Farnam Conolly, Georgia Hughes, Monique Muhlenkamp, Mary Ann Casler, and all the wonderful team of people at New World Library. Thank you for taking me by the hand and leading me through the amazing world of crafting a book. Thanks for your vision. Thanks for the hours of editing, designing, and creative juices poured into this work. Bill and I are forever grateful. And thank you for hooking me up with Eric Bolt.

To Eric Bolt, my developmental editor, thank you for the hours, days, weeks, and months of e-mails and phone calls aiding me along the journey of writing Bill's inspirational story. Thank you for cutting, pasting,

216

dressing up, and trimming down. Thank you for pushing me to pull stories locked inside and helping me express them in the best way possible.

I want to thank God for all of my many blessings including my friends and family mentioned and those not mentioned but in my heart. Most of all, I want to thank God whose hand, I believe, led our various paths to intersect. I am grateful to Him that my path crossed Bill Porter's so long ago. I am thankful that Bill hired me, didn't fire me, and eventually became my friend. Thank you, Bill, for your courageous, inspiring life. Thank you Bill, for being you.

The employees of Thorndike Press hope you have enjoyed this Large Print book. All our Thorndike and Wheeler Large Print titles are designed for easy reading, and all our books are made to last. Other Thorndike Press Large Print books are available at your library, through selected bookstores, or directly from us.

For information about titles, please call:

(800) 223-1244

or visit our Web site at:

www.gale.com/thorndike
www.gale.com/wheeler

To share your comments, please write:

Publisher
Thorndike Press
295 Kennedy Memorial Drive
Waterville, ME   04901

4445

PEACE

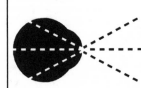

This Large Print Book carries the
Seal of Approval of N.A.V.H.

PEACE

RICHARD BAUSCH

THORNDIKE PRESS
A part of Gale, Cengage Learning

GALE
CENGAGE Learning·

Detroit • New York • San Francisco • New Haven, Conn • Waterville, Maine • London

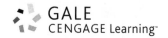

Copyright © 2008 by Richard Bausch.
Portions of this work originally appeared in *Narrative* magazine.
Thorndike Press, a part of Gale, Cengage Learning.

ALL RIGHTS RESERVED
This is a work of fiction. Names, characters, places, and incidents either are the product of the author's imagination or are used fictitiously. Any resemblance to actual persons, living or dead, events, or locales is entirely coincidental.
Thorndike Press® Large Print Historical Fiction.
The text of this Large Print edition is unabridged.
Other aspects of the book may vary from the original edition.
Set in 16 pt. Plantin.
Printed on permanent paper.

LIBRARY OF CONGRESS CATALOGING-IN-PUBLICATION DATA

Bausch, Richard, 1945–
  Peace / by Richard Bausch.
    p. cm. — (Thorndike Press large print historical fiction)
  ISBN-13: 978-1-4104-1170-9 (hardcover : alk. paper)
  ISBN-10: 1-4104-1170-2 (hardcover : alk. paper)
    1. World War, 1939–1945—Fiction. 2. Italy—Fiction. 3. Large
type books. I. Title.
  PS3552.A846P43 2008b
  813'.54—dc22   2008037782

Published in 2008 by arrangement with Alfred A. Knopf, Inc.

Printed in the United States of America
1 2 3 4 5 6 7 12 11 10 09 08

With love, for
ANN MARIE BAUSCH *and* WESLEY
BAUSCH,
who read these pages first

And in loving memory of my father,
ROBERT CARL BAUSCH,
who served bravely in Africa,
Sicily, and Italy

Lo, the moon ascending,
Up from the east the silvery
round moon,
Beautiful . . .

And my heart, O my soldiers,
my veterans,
My heart gives you love.
— WALT WHITMAN
"Dirge for Two Veterans," Drum Taps

With deepest gratitude, love, and admiration to George Garrett, who for almost twenty years kept after me to write this story

ONE

They went on anyway, putting one foot in front of the other, holding their carbines barrel down to keep the water out, trying, in their misery and confusion — and their exhaustion — to remain watchful. This was the fourth straight day of rain — a windless, freezing downpour without any slight variation of itself. Rivulets of ice formed in the muck of the road and made the walking treacherous. The muscles of their legs burned and shuddered, and none of them could get enough air. Robert Marson thought about how they were all witnesses. And nobody could look anybody in the eye. They kept on, and were punished as they went. Ice glazed their helmets, stuck to the collars of their field jackets, and the rain got in everywhere, soaking them to the bone. They were somewhere near Cassino, but it was hard to believe it was even Italy anymore. They had stumbled blind

11

into some province of drenching cold, a berg of death. Everything was in question now.

The Italians had quit, and the Germans were retreating, engaging in delaying actions, giving way slowly, skirmishing, seeking to make every inch of ground costly in time and in blood, and there were reconnaissance patrols all along the front, pushing north, heading into the uncertainty of where the Germans might be running, or waiting.

Marson, sick to his soul, barely matched the pace of the two men just in front of him, who were new. Their names were Lockhart and McCaig, and they themselves lagged behind four others: Troutman, Asch, Joyner, and Sergeant Glick. Seven men. Six witnesses.

The orders had been to keep going until you found the enemy. Then you were supposed to make your way back, preferably without having been seen. But the enemy had the same kinds of patrols, and so recon also meant going forward until you were fired upon. Worse, this was a foot patrol. If you ran into anything serious, there wouldn't be any jeeps to ride out, nor tanks to help you. You were alone in the waste of the war.

And there were only the seven of them now.

Twelve men had left one tank battalion the first day, crossed country, and then slept under the tanks of another on the second, all in the changeless fall of the rain. McConnell, Padruc, and Bailey came down with the dysentery and had to be taken back to Naples. So the patrol left that camp with nine men.

Walberg and Hopewell were killed yesterday.

Yesterday, a farmer's cart full of wet straw had come straggling along the road being pulled by a donkey and driven by two Italian boys — gypsies, really — who looked like sopping girls, their long, black, soaked hair framing their faces, their wet cloaks hiding their bodies. Sergeant Glick waved them away, and they melted into the glazed second growth beside the road. Then he ordered that the cart be overturned in order to look for weapons or contraband. Troutman and Asch accomplished this, and as the waterlogged, mud-darkened straw collapsed from the bed of the cart, a Kraut officer and a whore tumbled out, cursing. The Kraut shot Walberg and Hopewell with his black Luger before Corporal Marson put him down. The whore, soggy and dirty and ill looking, wearing another officer's tunic over a brown skirt, spoke only German, and she shouted more curses at them, gesticulating and trying to hit at McCaig and Joyner, who held her. And Sergeant Glick looked at Hopewell and Walberg, ascertained that they were dead, then walked over, put the end of his carbine at her forehead, and fired. The shot stopped the sound of her. She fell back into the tall wet stalks of grass by the side of the road, so that only her lower legs and her feet showed. She went over backward; the legs came up and then dropped with a thud into the sudden silence. Marson, who had been looking at the Kraut he shot, heard the fourth shot and turned to see this. And he saw the curve of her calves, the feet in a man's boots where they jutted from the grass. For a few seconds, no one said anything. They all stood silent and did not look at one another, or at Glick, and the only sound was the rain.

"She was with him. She'd've shot us all if she could," Glick said. No one answered him. Marson had shot the Kraut, and he was having trouble with that, and here were the woman's legs stuck out of the grass next to the road. The curve of the calves was that

14

of a young woman. "This is all one thing," Glick said, loud. It was as if he were talking to the earth and sky. The others knew he meant that the woman had been a reaction, two men killed like that — shot, both of them, through the heart — completely unready for it, though Glick had repeatedly told them and they all knew that they should be ready, every second, for just this. This. Walberg and Hopewell, two boys. Hopewell had just been talking about being at a restaurant in Miami Beach, eating Dungeness crabs, how much he wished he were there right now. And Walberg, quiet Walberg, only this morning had been going on about his father, who was a hero to him, and the others had been embarrassed hearing him describe the old man, because of the childlike devotion in it, the hero worship. "Grow up, Walberg," Asch had said once. And Walberg had grown up to this, lying by the side of a road somewhere near Cassino, with an expression on his face of mild surprise. Hopewell's eyes were closed. He looked like he was asleep.

And they had all been warned to be ready, every second.

But it had been so cold, and the rain kept coming down on them. They had got numb, maybe even drowsy — the drowse before you lie down and freeze to death. And they couldn't really look at one another now, and still nobody looked at Glick.

Because this was a recon squad — and because the Germans had taken over everything, the war and the retreat and the defense of Italy, and could be close — they had to leave Walberg and Hopewell beside the road and move on, away from the scene, while light left the low, charred-looking folds of the sky. Troutman had radioed back.

There had followed an abysmal long night without any respite from the cold and the rain. Through it all, nobody spoke of what had taken place back down the road. But Marson kept feeling the sickness. It was as if something in him had been leveled, and the simplest memories of himself as he had always been were beside the point. He was devout, because his people were devout, and because it was a strength, and he kept trying to pray, kept saying the words in his mind. *All for thee, most sacred heart of Jesus.* An offering, as he had been taught. Expiation for his sins, for everything he had ever done that was wrong. It meant little, now. At times he would speak directly to God in his mind, like a man talking to another man — except that it was somehow more than one other man or, really, one god; but

16

something nameless and immense beyond the raining sky: *Let me get through this, help me find forgiveness, and I'll raise a big family.* He had a daughter back home, a thirteen-month-old girl whom he had yet to see in person. He kept her photograph tucked away under his shirt, in a flat cigarette tin.

He could not let himself think very much at all. The others were quiet, sullen, isolated. And yet after the misery of the fitful night, they seemed to have put it in its place. It was the war; it was what they had been through. They had lived with confusion for so long. Nobody said anything about it.

They just slogged on, always north. And the sickness kept coming over Marson in waves. He had been on the beachhead at Salerno. His company had been pinned down for hours leading into days, and he had lived through the panic when all along the line men believed that the enemy had infiltrated the ranks, and they froze on their weapons and shot members of their own outfit who had gone beyond them. He had fired mortar rounds into the roil and tumult of the fortifications beyond the beach, had been in the fighting all the way to Persano and the Sele River, and he knew intellectually that he had certainly killed several men.

He had seen so much death, and the dead

17

no longer caused quite the same shock. Not even poor Walberg and Hopewell. He had experienced that kind of sudden stop before now. But he hadn't, himself, until yesterday, killed anyone up close. The Kraut had a big round boy's face and bright red hair, and the bullet had gone into him just above the breastbone and exited with a blast of blood and flesh out the back of his neck, into the distance behind him. He coughed bright blood mixed with something he must've had to eat, looking right at Corporal Marson with an expression terrifyingly like wonder, while the light or the animation or whatever it was left his green eyes, and the eyes started to reflect the raining sky, the clear, icy water gathering in them and running down the white face.

Two

Sunny Italy, John Glick had been calling it, spitting the words out, the standard joke in the lines. He was from New York and had worked as a longshoreman for a year out of high school, and you could hear it in his voice.

Four straight days of rain. It felt like the end of the world. The North Atlantic had gone up into the sky and traveled south and was coming down with temperatures wavering at the freezing point.

At early dusk today, another tank battalion caught up with them. They got under the tanks and ate rations, coughing and sputtering. Glick went a few paces down the row of tanks and half-tracks and reported about Walberg and Hopewell, the Kraut and the woman. Marson heard him say that she had been killed in the cross fire. He saw Joyner hear it, too, and Joyner looked at him, but then looked away. Nobody else in this battalion had run into any action yesterday, though Marson, crossing to the far side of the range of tanks and other equipment, encountered a soldier they had all talked to several days before, and he was sitting in the back of a jeep, holding his hand and crying. The hand had been burned badly; it was black and two of the fingers looked like charred twigs, and it was shaking as with a palsy. The soldier kept staring at it, crying like a little kid. No one could talk to him.

Marson gave forth a little sobbing breath, and turned away.

It was for what was called his steadiness on the beachhead at Salerno that he had been given a field promotion to corporal. The promoting officer used the word. Marson's company had been held down by machine-gun fire, and he had bolted forward to a shell crater in the sand and then lobbed grenades at the emplacement. Others had followed him, and the enemy withdrew, abandoning their own machine gun. There had been no time to think and in his memory of it, it was like trying to stop a leak in a seawall, shouting all the time. Marson had felt no steadiness, but only the sense of trying very hard not to die, and the frozen conviction at his middle that he would not survive the next minute. He was older than most of these boys, twenty-six. It astonished him that so many of them believed that they could not die. Even seeing death on the beach at Salerno.

Now he and Joyner sat in a mired jeep briefly to get out of the rain. They did not particularly like each other. There had been tension between them before. Joyner had a set of attitudes about Negroes, Jews, and Catholics, and his assertions, along with the obscenity of his speech in general, had an unpleasant air of authority about them, as if he had done serious study and come to serious conclusions. But it all came from ignorance and bigotry. Joyner, apparently sensing the effect on Marson, claimed he was joking. But for Marson the jokes were seldom very clever, or very funny, and it was unnerving. He had, to his great discomfort, discerned the thinnest echo of his own casually held assumptions in the other man's talk. And so he had worked to keep a distance.

Until now.

He had seen the look Joyner gave him when Sergeant Glick spoke of the whore's death. So, sitting behind the driver's wheel of the jeep, he had the sense that he ought to see if Joyner, given the chance, might say something. Except that he was too honest with himself to believe this was the only motive: the truth was that he wanted to learn what all the others felt. He was too muddled and tired to think clearly enough. But he wanted to know.

Joyner did not disappoint him. Watching him light a cigarette and blow the smoke, he muttered: "Some cross fire, huh?"

Marson looked over at him and then looked away. It came to him that he did not want to talk about it with Joyner. Not with him.

"Cross fire like that and you don't need a fuck'n firing squad," Joyner went on, smiling, spitting from between his teeth, a habit he had. He was tall and narrow eyed, with a long nose and big, wide-fingered hands that always shook. He had once talked of how it was a problem lighting a lady's cigarette. And he had sworn it wasn't nerves. He had a recurring itch on his left forearm. That, he said, *was* nerves, since he'd never had anything like it until the war. It was always there, since Sicily, and he kept having to dig at it.

They sat together in the front seat of the jeep, which was up to its axle in the mud of the road and was therefore out of the war for now. They did not quite look at each other. Marson drew on the cigarette.

"I thought Salerno was fucked up," Joyner said, scratching the place on his forearm.

At Salerno, he had been entrenched with several others near a crippled LCI that rolled back and forth in the heavy waves behind them. They heard the loud pinging of bullets hitting the metal of the LCI, and Joyner kept up a stream of obscenities. It made a strange undersound to the crackle of the firing and the waves pounding, the planes going over and the bombs falling, and the high whistle of the ordnance coming from the ships at the horizon line, and the screams of those who had been hit. Finally he broke from the trench and came running. He crossed a wide rib of sand and ossified wood and dropped down next to a corpsman, who fell in the next instant, helmet breaking with the metal clank of the bullet or fragment that killed him. Joyner fired at the culvert above them and kept firing. Then he screamed. "Fuck!" It went off in a falsetto shriek. And that was when the realization came to them all that the firing from the culvert had all but ceased.

They rushed it, and overran it, and found that after days of delivering a withering fire, the enemy had withdrawn. Joyner sat against the seawall and wept like a baby, mouth agape, eyes closed, the tears running.

Now, sitting with him in the jeep in the pelting rain, smoking the cigarette, the corporal remembered this pass and kept his eyes averted.

"I don't give a shit about it," Joyner said suddenly. "You know that, right?"

Marson offered him a drag of the cigarette.

"Fuck you."

"Just trying to keep the peace, there, Joyner."

"Yeah. Peace. Would you have tried to stop it?"

"I didn't see it happen. I heard it and looked."

"That isn't what I asked you."

"The answer is, I don't know. Okay? There wasn't a vote, you know. I don't think anybody could've done anything."

"You're white as a sheet."

Marson took a drag of the cigarette and did not answer. They were quiet for a little while.

"You look like all hell."

"What would you have done?" Marson asked him. "Would you have tried to stop it?"

"Fuck," Joyner said. "I'd've shot her myself. But I wouldn't have called it a fuck'n cross fire."

Marson felt the sickness. But he could not tell this to Joyner or show it to him.

"This rain is the fuck'n end-times," Joyner said abruptly. "The end of the fuck'n world."

"It's rain," said the corporal.

"I'm telling you I never saw four straight goddamn days of fuck'n ice falling from the fuck'n sky."

Sergeant Glick came back past the line of tanks. "Fall in," he said. He'd been given five new troops. He ordered them to say their names. They stood on either side of him, like the members of a posse. They looked weary and aggravated, muttering their own names. Phillips, Carrick, Dorfman, Bruce, Nyman.

"The Jerries are still rolling back," Glick said. "But they're leaving stragglers, for attrition. You all get that?"

The men made a general low sound of agreement.

"There's snipers and combat patrols out there, looking to make us miserable."

"Mission already accomplished," said Asch. A couple of the new men laughed.

"If you don't want to die," Glick said, "you'll keep your eyes peeled and your weapons ready and your ears open."

"Got a back problem, Sergeant," Asch said.

25

"Should've had it looked at Stateside," Glick said. But he knew what was coming.

"Nobody would do a thing about it."

"That's tough."

"Yeah, Sarge."

"Cut it out, Asch."

"Yeah, trouble is, I got a big wide yellow streak right down the middle of it."

"Asch, I might have you court-martialed just for your mouth."

"Watch for those snipers, Sarge."

THREE

They all headed out, still north, still on foot. The road was deep mud, turning to ice, grabbing at their feet, and the rain kept coming — straight down, relentless, pitiless, miserable. At some point during today's march, Marson had developed a blister on his right heel. Some inconsistency or tear in the leather of the insole in his boot hurt him with each step, and each step made it worse, and the sickness was still with him.

The pain went up to his ankle, shooting, like nerve pain. There wasn't any way to favor it. Even limping seemed to give no relief. And each time the images of what happened on the road came to him — Walberg and Hopewell lying so still; the woman's legs jutting from the grass; the green eyes of the soldier he had shot, reflecting light, the look of wonder in the white face — each time these things went through him, his gorge rose. But then, in the freezing minutes turning into hours that went on, and on, he found himself realizing that this shock, like all the others, was fading, too. And there was just the constant, hollow presence of the nausea, along with the searing pain in his heel. Everyone was suffering a kind of low-grade shock, aware of the badness of being here, out of all the places there were to be in the world.

You marched into the tide of the war and arrived nowhere. Or you were among those who gave way to the lure of the war and rode off with a company of fools, looking for trouble. Asch trudged along next to him, muttering about the inadequacy of the army's version of a field jacket to keep out the rain and the cold. But then he leaned toward Marson and said, "We gotta do something."

Marson looked over at him, but said nothing.

"What are we, anyway?"

"Are you asking me?" Marson said.

Glick, a few yards ahead of them, turned and barked at a couple of the new troops: "Keep your distance, somebody'll get you both with one shot."

Asch dropped back a pace or two and moved to the right. He said, "My uncle's a police officer."

Marson glanced over at him.

"Homicide detective."

"Really."

"Twenty years."

Marson tried to adjust his stride to accommodate the pain in his heel and ankle. It was only getting worse.

"Do you ever wonder how somebody can do that all those years? One murder after another?"

"Never gave it any thought," Marson said.

"I never did, either, I guess. Until now."

Marson looked at him. "I know," he said. "It's a thought."

"Lot of them unsolved, too. Used to be kind of frustrating to him. The one thing he really hated was the people who could've helped him and wouldn't."

"Guess that would be hard."

"People who saw things and wouldn't say what they saw."

"Right."

"Yeah," Asch said. "Right."

"Did he ever figure what to do about it?"

"No."

"He still on the force?"

"Twenty years," Asch said.

Marson looked over at him. Asch was staring, his helmet pushed back, the rain splattering his face.

"You know what I mean?"

"That's a lot of years," Marson said.

"A lot of murders," said Asch.

Marson did not answer him this time. He experienced the nausea and the cold, and ahead of him the others were mechanically going on, shoulders hunched, the rain beating down on them, thin, falling strands of ice.

When they stopped to rest for a few minutes in the shell of a farmhouse, he worked to get his boot off to try doing something about the foot. But it was the shape of the heel itself, something pushing upward from the insole, a wrinkle. The foot looked whiter than could be healthy, except for the place where the blister bulged. He broke it with the point of his bayonet and let it run, and the flap of skin, about the size of a quarter, collapsed into the redness, the inflamed center of the abrasion. It hurt to touch it. He let the rain pelt it as long as he could, until the sting was too much, and then he put the sock back on — it was wet through, and heavy — and the boot, hurting, trying to offer up the pain, trying to think in terms of the prayer. *All for thee.* The foot throbbed, and there was the problem of the cold now, too, and the marching went on, and each time he put the weight of himself on the foot, the pain shot up to his ankle, a piercing white-hot flash. He winced at it and went on, and suffered it. A flatness had settled into his spirit, a dead feeling at the heart. It was as if the physical pain could have been happening to someone else. It did not reach into him, quite. There was something removed at the very center, and he could turn in his mind and look at the empty place.

FOUR

Toward sundown, they stopped where a fast-moving river came up to the edge of the road on the left and went on, veering off again into the trees. The road wound sharply to the right and out of sight beyond the rise of a steep hill. There were trees on that side, too. Through the trees to the left was the water, metal gray and solid looking, with little quick flags of white in it. Now and again a tree branch came gliding past, and then they saw boards and other debris, followed by the legs of a horse, the animal being pulled along in the swirling eddies, bobbing in and out of the folds of water, the legs frozen in an attitude of flight. The river churned and roared. They all moved to the right of the road and the base of the hill, where the wet black branches provided some meager shelter. All the trees were beginning to look as though they were made of glass. There were tank tracks in the mud and stones of the road. Glick had Troutman bring the radio to him and reported this, and they all waited. There wasn't any sound but the rain coming down. The word came through to keep going.

But Glick didn't move. The others watched him. Little slivers of ice dropped down off his helmet. It took another moment for them to realize that he had seen something coming from the bend of the road. It was another farm cart, this one being pulled by a horse. A crooked shape in brown, a hooded man with dark thin hands, held the reins. Under the hood was only the suggestion of a gaunt face in shadow. The cart came abreast of them, and Glick rushed it, his carbine at the ready. The figure stopped the cart and stood in it, hands up. It was an old man. He looked at them wide eyed and spoke in a trembling reedy voice. "*Sono italiano.* Speaka English." Then in Italian again: "*Non sono tedesco! Amico, sono il vostro amico. Amico. Non uccidermi! Non spararmi! Per favore!* No shoot."

"You *capeesh* English?" Glick said to him.

"*Poco,*" the old man said through a wide grimace that showed broken and decayed teeth. "*Sì, un po'.* Little. Speaka the English. Little. *Sì.*"

"Get down off the cart."

He hesitated, looking at them all, plainly unsure of what was being asked and fearing that any miscalculation would be the end of him. Then: *"Cedo! Non spararmi!* Surrender! No shoot, *per favore."*

"Down," Glick said, gesturing. "Get the fuck down."

The rain on the old man's lined, bony face made it look as though he was crying. His eyes were squeezed tight, the brows pinched. It was a look of great sorrow. Glick motioned with the end of the rifle. "Now," he said. And with alacrity, evidently trying desperately to please, the old man climbed down.

Glick got Lockhart to unhitch the horse and then ordered Joyner and Troutman to upset the cart while the others crouched, ready to fire. He instructed Marson to cover the old man, who stood there quietly with the rain beating down on him, the cowl-like hood obscuring much of his face. The cloak he wore was made of the same canvas material that was stretched over whatever was in the cart. He wore rope-soled shoes, and his pants were thick burlap, drooping past the ankles, mud stained and wet to the knees. The look of him was of a kind of sad resignation — here was his cart, with all his

34

belongings in it, being overturned in the road. The cart contained nothing but the possessions of somebody trying to ride with his little life away from a war. Marson thought of the old man's humiliation: shoes and dishes and pictures of family members, clothes, books, cooking utensils. The old man turned away slightly, as if the sight of these things hurt him.

"You know this country?" Glick asked him, *"Capeesh?"* He made a motion to include the trees and the tall hill, the sodden surroundings.

"Si, si."

"Guide? Scout?" Glick turned and pointed up the hill into the trees.

"Scout." The man simply repeated the word.

Glick pointed at the bend in the road. "German?"

The old man nodded, but it was impossible to tell whether he meant that he understood or that there were Jerries up the road. He stood there with that look of resignation and watched the rain collect in the little folds of his thrown clothing and on his belongings lying in the mud.

"Set the cart right," Glick told the others. "Put his stuff back. Marson, keep your rifle on him."

The others did as they were told. For Marson, it felt for a moment all right, even with the general terror, the pain, and the shivering. It was a correction. The old man watched them.

"You guide?" Glick said, pointing up into the trees.

The man stared at him.

"Go up over fucking hill," Glick said with exaggerated slowness, pointing. "Christ sakes. See fucking road. Get it? Over the fucking hill, see the fucking road."

Marson indicated himself, and then the old man, and then the hill rising behind him. "Guide," he said.

"Oh, *sì. Sì. Vi guiderò. Sì,* yes."

"*Guiderò.* Guide," Glick said.

"Yes. *Sì.*"

He turned to Marson. "Take Asch and Joyner."

The old man waited, turning slightly. The sergeant ordered the cart pulled off the road, into the trees by the river. The horse had been tied to one of the trees there, and it stood watching them all, blinking in the rain but apparently not even quite noticing it, tearing at the grass at the base of the tree and chewing, staring. The blanket over its haunches had gone black with soaking, and it gave off a stream of little silver turning-

36

to-ice drops.

"Now," Glick said. "Goddamn. What're you waiting for? Move it."

The old man nodded, then turned to Marson and motioned for him to follow. Marson thought he saw something of a smile on the wet, drawn, aged features. A look of relief, he realized.

"Asch," he said. "Joyner."

The two troops fell in line and they started up into the trees, the old man leading the way.

FIVE

It was slow going. The hill became steadily steeper, and it was slippery. A thick bed of pine needles and mud and dead leaves covered the ground. They had to dig with the toes of their boots to make footholds in it. They hadn't gone fifty yards before Asch fell and slipped back, and he made a sound like a yelp, an animal noise. He had hit the trunk of a tree on the way down. He had been stopped by it.

Marson, Joyner, and the old man waited for him to get up. They were still in sight of the others on the road, who were now resting in the failing light, huddled in the torrent, the relentless emptying sky.

"Christ, why us?" Joyner said, to no one in particular.

They waited, and Asch fell again, cursing.

"Shit sakes, Asch," Joyner said.

The old man had paused, one leg up, ready to keep on, and his face was impassive, merely interested in Asch's progress climbing back to them. At one point, Asch went to his knees and stayed there, his face contorted with the effort and with the frustration of not being able to gain his footing. But then his expression changed. He sighed and leaned forward and rested his arms on the barrel of his carbine. He seemed almost content, kneeling there while they gazed down at him, perhaps twenty yards farther up.

"Come on, asshole," Joyner said.

"Fuck you," said Asch.

Marson thought he heard Joyner say something under his breath. He believed he had heard the word *Yid.* He looked at Joyner, who had pulled a rag out of his field jacket and was wiping his face.

"You'd best keep your opinions to yourself," he said.

Joyner folded the rag and put it away and then merely stared.

"Got it?" Marson said.

"I *capeesh,*" said Joyner. "What're you gonna do, fire me?"

Asch got to them and then dropped to his knees again, having slipped and stopped himself. He turned and looked back down at the road. "I'm shorter than you guys. It's harder to climb. Don't go so fast."

"We don't have all night," the corporal said.

"You think they're above us? Waiting up there?" Asch wanted to know.

"How the fuck would we have that information," said Joyner.

"Just keep alert," Marson told them.

"Going down this fucker isn't going to be much easier than going up if we have to move quick," Asch said. "I really hit my back on that sapling going down. Can we take a minute? It really hurts."

"Maybe you should head on back down, darling," Joyner said. "We wouldn't want you to get a boo-boo."

"Fuck yourself," Asch told him. "Better yet, why don't you stand up real straight, and then fall through your asshole and hang yourself?"

"Bright boy," Joyner said. "All you New York guys are so bright."

"Shut up," Marson said.

"All of *what* guys, Joyner. You want to give me a more specific category? I happen to be from Boston."

"You know what category."

"I don't have any idea, buddy. Why don't you fill me in?"

Joyner said nothing.

The old man stood there watching them

40

with that expression of calm interest. When he saw Corporal Marson looking at him, he straightened slightly and pulled his own cloak higher around his neck.

"We're going to make this walk to the top of this hill and see what we can see," Marson said. "And then we're going to turn around and come back down, and we are not going to waste any energy fighting with each other. Got it?"

"I fell," Asch said. "Jesus. Tell him to lay off."

"No, I'm not getting between you. I'm telling you both how it's gonna be."

"You want to tell him to lay off the New York stuff? Because that's not what he means."

Marson looked at Joyner, who had a challenge in his eyes. The rain was making him blink, but his eyes were cold and defiant. "You didn't mean that like it sounded, right, Joyner?"

"Could've been talking about any big city," Joyner said.

"Fuck you," said Asch. "No matter what you were talking about."

The old man murmured something low.

"No *capeesh,*" Joyner said to him. "Did you say you want us to die choking on our own blood?"

The old man simply returned his gaze.

"This is a fuck'n Fascist, I'm telling you," Joyner said.

"Non sono fascista," said the old man, with an earnest shaking of his head. He began to wring his old hands. It looked like he was trying to bend the bones in them.

"Now you've spooked him," Marson said. "Keep your mouth shut, Joyner. Just don't open it again."

Asch got to his feet. "I'm ready when you are," he said to Marson.

They turned and started up, following the path where the old man led them, still struggling with the steep angle of the hill and the slippery surface, with its little rushing trickles of water, the rain still beating down with the same windless fall.

"Oh, Christ," Joyner said. "Why does it have to be us?"

Six

Joyner was from Michigan, a sheep farm there, where his father and grandfather and great-grandfather had lived; and his father had raised him to take over, in time. The war was his escape, as he had told anyone who would listen in the first days they all were together. He hated the farm — hated the *idea* of farming — and spent much of his time in high school following the good orchestras around the upper Midwest. He played clarinet, and his father thought of him as a bum, he said, and that was a tough thing to live with sometimes. He had once seen Benny Goodman at the Aragon Ballroom in Chicago, and he talked about the women he met that night and about walking along the lake in the summer dark with the city shining on the water. He could be expressive in that way, too, which made him all the more troublesome to Marson, who was himself expressive and liked what his mother always called *picture speech,* words and phrases that took you somewhere other than where you were. Joyner said that he liked Benny Goodman best because his own name was Benny, and then he went on to say that a coincidence of naming was no reason to like a man's music, either. But there it was.

And there Joyner was. He could talk about the moon shining on water, and yet obscenity flowed from him like the little beads of spit he kept throwing off. He would spray it out from between his teeth. This punctuated his talk, like a nerve-tic.

In Palermo, in training, he would look up and see Marson coming, and, knowing of Marson's reluctance to use bad language, he would spit and say, "Aw fuck-shit. I mean gosh." Others found it funny, including Asch, but it made Marson feel singled out.

"I got off the fuck'n farm and here I am in farm country, in fuck'n Italy," Joyner would say. It was as though he were reciting it.

"You should've brought your clarinet," Marson told him once, trying not to show how awkward he felt. He had been a Benny Goodman fan, too, though he liked Glenn Miller better. He tried to shift the subject to music.

But Joyner brought it back to Marson's devoutness. "No atheists in the foxholes, right, Marson?"

"I guess not," Marson said.

"Fuck a duck, huh?"

And it was Asch who laughed. "Joyner, you should be on Broadway."

"Nothing for me in Jew York, there, Asch."

"On the curbside on Broadway, darling."

"Yeah, that's me all right, in that town. I'd have to stay drunk all the time."

"Hey, I've got an idea, how about you kiss my ass?"

Like Marson, Joyner had been a star athlete in high school — right guard on the football team, forward on the basketball team. He played baseball, too, but wasn't as good at it, nor as interested in it. Marson had been so good at baseball that he played semipro for a couple of years. He had been around. He was the oldest man in the squad, two years older than Sergeant Glick. Joyner was only nineteen. He and Marson had come through training together. They were assigned to the division when it was still in Sicily, following the invasion there. Saul Asch had seen action in North Africa and he talked about a dream he kept having from a memory: a burning tank, the men in it, and the heat of the desert, the smell rising in the waves of black smoke and flames. He dreamed the smell, he said, and his tone was matter-of-fact, as though he were reporting some curiosity of the terrain. The dream did not appear to affect him. He was just twenty-three years old, with round little brown eyes and chubby boy's cheeks, the eldest of three brothers, all of whom were serving. He had barely made the height requirement. Marson had found him pleasurable to be around because of the way he had of turning everything into an observation, and there was the Boston accent. But he had lately been wanting to avoid him because of his talk about the recurring dream. It kept happening. "Had it again," he would say. "Same thing. The heat and the smell. Like I'm there again." He would shake his head and shrug. "You figure?" That was a phrase he used repeatedly to express puzzlement or wonder. He was Jewish, but, as he put it, never practiced. His grandfather was a German Jew who in his late thirties fought for the Kaiser in World War I. That always amazed him to think about. The grandfather had died last year in the living room of an apartment in Brockton, after eating a meal of salmon in dill sauce with his daughter-in-law, who had cooked the meal and came from Italy. That man had been in the other war, the first one, fighting on the other side. Asch talked about going from the Ardennes Forest, shooting at French and English and American soldiers, to a living room in Brockton — with a grandson about to join the army to go fight the Hun. It was ridiculous.

Marson possessed a strong sense of paradox, and he had liked this story. But he had been having trouble being around Asch: he would think of it, and of the Africa nightmare, every time Asch spoke. It was like backdrop. And now they had the woman's death between them, too.

Marson couldn't imagine Asch living long enough to be a grandfather. Probably it was the rounded cheeks, so boylike, so chubby and smooth. Marson couldn't look at him without thinking that the war would certainly kill him. But then, often he did not, himself, expect to survive it.

Seven

It was almost full dark now. The cold was a dead immensity on them. It was as though they were moving through a film of ice, always climbing, weighted down by web belt and pack, and the bandoliers and grenades, slipping, fighting for air, following the old man, who seemed to have grown younger as the distance between him and the road increased. He climbed easily, and his breathing seemed effortless. Marson watched him, his own lungs burning, his legs trembling with the effort not to fall. The climb kept getting steeper, and he could hear his own heart pounding in his ears. He gagged, and then gagged again, climbing. Each step scraped the blister on his heel, and several times he had to use the stock of his rifle like a cane, the palm of his hand over the barrel opening, to support himself. Asch and Joyner were silent, and they made no eye contact, automatically thrusting themselves up with each step, using a tree branch now and then to pull on. They came up, oblivious to anything but the slant of the ground where they were putting their boots — the rough angling upward of the earth with its rucks and broken branches and gouges of mud and leaf meal — and Marson kept looking back at them, checking their progress. It was too dark now to see where they were heading or where the hill might begin to crest or level off. There was just the endless climbing, pain deepening in the muscles of their legs and in their knees, the bones there. Because the ground was so steep, there didn't seem to be a way to rest without beginning the long slide back down. And all the while there was the unabating, remorseless, utter constancy of the rain.

The old man went on up, the incline so steep now that with each step that knee was close to his chest, the bony hand pushing on it, to gain the next increment of ground. Asch fell again and slid far enough to be out of sight. Joyner sat down and put the butt of his rifle against the ground between his feet, his field jacket sleeve across the barrel. He reached in under the sleeve and scratched the place on his forearm. Marson called softly to the old man. "Wait."

"*Si.*"

The old man held on to the thin trunk of a tree, and Marson climbed to him, then turned. They could hear Asch struggling toward them from where he had fallen.

"*Che città* in America?" the old man said. "City you live?"

"Washington, D.C.," Marson said.

"I see Washington."

"Yeah?"

Silence. Just the clink of equipment on the belts, the rain beating their bodies and the helmets. Above them, the sky was inconsistently covering a full moon — there were thin places in it — but the rain kept beating down. The old man wiped the water from his chin and coughed. Then he bent a little at his knees, reached into his burlap trousers, and pulled out his prick. In the dimness, Marson saw the uncircumcised length of it. The old man urinated onto the soggy leaves at his feet. The urine steamed, running in thin tributaries away from him. He tucked himself back in and, looking at Marson, nodded slightly, with an embarrassed little smile.

"When did you see Washington?" Marson asked him.

After a hesitation, the old man nodded. "Younger. I travel. *Sono andato a* New York. I — I go to New York, too. Yes?"

"Yes," Marson told him. "I've never been."

The old man seemed mystified.

"No me," Marson said. "New York."

"Ah, *sì*."

"What is your name?"

Again the look.

"How are you called?"

The old man nodded. "Yes. *Sì*."

Marson pointed to himself. "Robert."

"*Sì*. Angelo."

"Angelo."

"Were you ever in the army, Angelo?"

"Come?"

Marson pointed to himself, his helmet with the water dripping from it. "Army. Military."

"Oh, *sì. Nella prima guerra*."

"*Prima*. One. World War I."

"*Sì*."

"Did you fight?"

The old man stared.

"Fight." Marson gestured, pantomimed shooting.

"*Sì. Ero un capitano*."

Marson saluted him. "Captain, *sì*?"

The old man, Angelo, nodded. He had a hopeful expression on his face now. Water dripped from the creases of his hood and gathered at his chest, the large fold there. The rain got in. It ran searchingly down

Marson's neck and into his blouse. He shivered. Asch made it to them, and finally they all headed up again, reaching for crevices and low branches because it was too steep to stand. The ground kept sliding beneath them, and the icy rain kept pelting their faces.

At last they came to a small area of level ground, and Marson said, "We'll rest here a little."

Angelo looked at him.

"Rest?" Marson said again.

"*Sì.*"

Asch and Joyner were already pulling their packs off. They set them down and, with their rifles across their thighs, squatted against an outcropping of rock, a ledge that channeled the rain away from them, down the mountain. It was a mountain. Marson realized that now. The old man moved to the ledge, to Asch's left. Marson joined him there. They were all four huddled in the lee of the rock, and the water ran on away from them, though Marson's knees were still exposed. He took his blanket roll and opened it and held it over himself.

"Fuck," Asch said. "When I get out of this, I'm gonna live in the desert, I swear to Christ. I'm gonna move to Arizona. And if it rains *there* I'm moving. I'm gonna be somewhere in the sun." He sounded as though he might start shrieking.

"Keep it down," Marson told him. He almost choked on the words. The muscles of his abdomen contracted. He swallowed and took a slow breath. They were all quiet, hearing the noise of the rain that kept coming and coming.

"I'm telling you it's the end of the fucking world," Joyner said. "The world never had to deal with so much general destruction. How do we know we won't knock it right off its orbit into space?"

"Jesus, Ben. I got enough morbid shit running around in my head without worrying about *that,* too."

"Don't call me Ben. It's Benny."

"Sorry there, Joyner."

"Christ," Joyner said. "I never even got married." He put his hand in under his sleeve and scratched again.

"Wonder if my wife's had her baby," said Asch. Then, after clearing his throat: "I don't think a woman should die because she's got blood loyalty to a lover." He cleared his throat again, and bowed his head and spit. "Christ's sake."

"Saint Saul," Joyner said. "Maybe you didn't notice she was trying to claw my fuck'n eyes out."

"I noticed. I notice everything, buddy."

"Is that some kind of threat?"

"Shut it," Corporal Marson said. "Both of you."

Joyner turned to him. "You think anybody else is out in this shit, Marson?"

"If they are, and they're Jerries, they'll have weapons, too," Marson told him. "So shut it."

"I'm shivering so bad," Asch muttered. "I've got cramps from the shivering. I hit my back on a sapling, sliding down the fucking hill."

"It's not a hill," Joyner said, scratching. "It's a fuck'n mountain."

"Mountain, *sì,*" said the old man. *"Montagna."*

"This is bullshit, is what this is."

"Shut up," Corporal Marson said. "All of you."

They were quiet again. He looked out at the faintly glistening tree and branch shapes in the dark and listened to the rain, its amazing monotonous drumming. He closed his eyes and saw again the softly curved dirty legs of the woman jutting from the tall drenched grass and the Kraut with his dying green eyes, such a dark shade of green, and the red hair matted to the white forehead. That look of pure wonder. Something

54

like a thrill went through him, horrible, and then inexpressible, gone, a feather's touch in his soul, like something reaching for him from the bottom of hell. He looked at the others there with him in the raining dark and was afraid for them, not thinking of himself at all, and it was as if he had already died, and saw them from some other plane of existence.

"Avete da mangiare?" the old man murmured. "Eat? Food."

Marson opened a tin of C rations and handed it to him. He ate greedily, with his fingers, as if wanting to get it down before it could be taken away from him.

The others ate, too, in silence. Marson could not do it. He smoked a cigarette and watched them, and then turned his head away. After a time, they were all trying to fall asleep. Marson closed his eyes again and almost immediately fell into a fitful slumber. He saw the old man sneak away into the mist that surrounded them, and then he was trying to stir himself. He heard breathing, voices murmuring, somebody said a name, or cursed, or commanded, and there was motion again and he couldn't break the spell, couldn't make the muscles of his arms or legs move. He was crying out now, in his dream, trying to get them to wake him.

Wake me up! he was shouting, and then he did stir, into a quiet, a stillness that brought him nearly to his feet, rifle held up, and he looked into the dark, and something moved. But there wasn't any movement and the only sound was the unceasing rain. He looked over and saw that the old man had curled up into his cloak and gone to sleep. The other two were also asleep, Asch with his helmet almost off and his fat cheeks twitching. Asch was probably dreaming of Africa again. "No," he said once, loud. And then again: "No."

EIGHT

Robert Marson had arrived in Palermo on a troopship after the initial fighting there was over. And there had been some delays about further orders. In the area of the war in which he found himself, nobody seemed to know what to do with anybody. Many of them, it was rumored, would be part of an enormous operation somewhere along the coast of France. Others would go to the Italian mainland. They were all training and drilling for amphibious landings. Marson's unit was quartered in a row of pup tents on the outskirts of the city. The Tyrrhenian Sea was visible from their little strip of land. Out in the waters of the harbor there were minesweepers. But it was a peaceful, quiet scene. The idleness made everyone edgy. General Patton didn't want anybody getting too comfortable, or taking it too easy, and so they were performing drills through the early morning hours. But there were delays in deployment, and for a few days they had a kind of vacation. When there was any kind of break, they went into the city and to the beaches nearby and swam in the chilly water and sunned themselves on the sand. They felt an urgency about it all because they knew the war was waiting for them. In the lucid water of the sea, in the brightness and calm of the beach, it was difficult to believe in the war. Marson saw the Palatine Chapel and walked to a Norman castle with several other men.

In a little café off a square, within sight of a mosque, he drank several beers and then two bottles of wine with Saul Asch while Asch talked about his grandfather, the Kaiser's soldier. And about his parents, who were devout, and from whom he had kept his growing skepticism. "Sometimes," he said, "lies are better than truth. Trust me." Finally he began talking about his wife. A sweet woman. Fifteen years older than he. A teacher who had lived next door all through his growing up. "That's me, buddy. I married the lady next door. A widow, no less. You know how her husband died? Slipped in the bath. No kidding. Fell over and conked his head and that was that. He'd served us iced tea the afternoon it happened. Singing in the shower and the next minute: dead. It doesn't only take war, you know? I knew the guy, too. Nice guy. A little dull. Didn't talk much."

"Asch," Marson said. "You're the most morbid son of a bitch in this army."

"We're all in the crosshairs," Asch said. "That's all I know."

Marson told him about his wife and child. He wanted to try imagining himself to be somewhere after the war, wanted to place himself years away from it in his mind. He carried his wife's letters with him and the little cracked photo of the girl. His wife's name was Helen Louise. The baby's name was Barbara. He had not seen combat yet and he was afraid. He did not want to die or be wounded, of course, but he also feared that he would turn and run when the time came. These others all seemed so certain they would survive, and there were moments in the nights when he believed he would turn and run. He had read the Crane novel about the civil war, and Crane's conclusion — that his fictional soldier had seen the great death and it was, after all, only death — seemed utterly false to him, dangerously, stupidly romantic. He looked at Asch with these thoughts running in his mind and said the names of his wife and daughter, feeling the cold rising at the back of his head, the electric change in the nerves of his spine whenever he received the sense that he would not live to see his daughter or to look upon Helen's face again.

"Nice names," Asch said. "My wife's name is Clara. Sweet lady. When I'm thirty she'll be forty-five."

Marson looked at him.

"You figure?"

"It's more strange if you go the other way. How old was she when you were ten?" He was just talking to keep it all at bay, now.

"Yeah. Jesus," Asch said.

"A little boy."

"When I'm forty-five, she'll be sixty."

"We've got the arithmetic down," Marson said.

"You figure?"

"Fifteen years isn't really so much, is it?"

"Nothing to it, no. Just a thought, you know."

A dark boy came to the table, with a long thin face, beetle brows, a wide mouth, and a leonine shock of black hair. "This wine you're drinking is gutter water," he said, in clear unaccented English.

They were surprised. Marson smiled at him and the boy stared.

"You have a gap in your teeth."

Marson nodded, a little confused.

The boy pulled the skin of his wide mouth back, revealing that he had a missing front tooth. "We're meant to be friends, signore," he said, and introduced himself.

His name was Mario and he was from Messina. He had come to Palermo with his father and brother a year ago, and he knew where all the good wine was hidden. He went on to say that he could speak English so well because he had spent a summer in New York back when he was eight. He had spoken nothing but English that entire summer.

"New York," Asch said, "That's a big city. I'm from Boston."

"I confess I don't like Boston," the boy said. "The Dodgers play there."

"No, that's Brooklyn. Boston is the Red Sox."

"The hated Red Sox."

"My team," said Asch.

"I'm fucked to hear it. I am devoted to the New York Yankees."

"I hate the Yankees," Asch said. "And I hate everybody that likes them."

Mario smiled, showing the wide gap in his teeth. "Then we are sworn enemies, signore." At fifteen, he had yet to begin growing whiskers. He was lean, long limbed, and his hair was so black it showed blue. He

61

told them he had lost his tooth from getting pistol-whipped by a German soldier in Messina. The soldier hit him just for being dark skinned, swiping carelessly across his face with the barrel of the pistol. The boy described this with a smile as if it was all a very stupid joke. The soldier had been shot the next morning from the air by a strafing American plane that had a long-fanged mouth painted on the fuselage. Plenty of teeth in that mouth. Ten soldiers had died in the square from the one pass the plane made, and everybody was sure now that the Germans were through. "I will get you some good wine," he said. "The best wine. Primitivo."

"We'll pay for it," said Marson.

The boy went away and in less than an hour he returned with two bottles under his shirt. The wine was very dark and strong tasting, with a heavy aroma, and the flavor of it lingered on the tongue. It made Marson realize how bad the wine was that they had been drinking.

They were drunk coming back to the unit, and they slipped into their tents as if this were reconnaissance.

The fact was that the whole army seemed confused and not to know where its own soldiers were. There were also soldiers from the other armies — British and Canadian and free French — and there were many combinations of rank, including warrant officers and merchant seamen. Marson and Asch spent time with some of these others, talking about going home and about how maybe the war would end before they had to go where it was. On two other occasions they returned to the café, and each time Mario brought them the good wine.

Other soldiers went into the city and got into trouble. One soldier, a gunnery sergeant, stabbed a man over an Italian girl in one of the saloons. Several people witnessed it and they chased him down and beat him bloody like a dog in the street. The army was going to try him for attempted murder, but then lessened the charge to assault with a deadly weapon. Mario had all of the details.

There wasn't anything to do but unload the ships that kept coming into the harbor. The ships kept unloading troops, too, so the numbers kept getting bigger. There were times when the beaches were crowded, looking like the vacation beaches of home, except that there were very few women. But then the weather turned miserably hot, and several men contracted sandfly fever and malaria. Orders came, forbidding entry into the city anymore.

In the early mornings, in the increasing heat, they went through training and drilling. The first hot days of August were spent in discomfort and sweat work, followed by hours of enforced idleness.

Corporal Marson, halfway up the mountain in the freezing rain near Cassino, remembered how hot it had been in Palermo, and how much he had hated it.

They all hated the inactivity and the waiting and the living out of a pack, not to mention the first and most discouraging matter, being away from home. Home. The word had a resonance that could choke you, and Marson lay awake at night trying very hard not to allow it into his thoughts at all. The thinking itself was terrible. You always ended with the same ache. The idea of never seeing home again burned deep, and he would lie on his side with his knees up and try to pray. Rumors went through the ranks like infection — talk that the Italians would seek an armistice, and that this might truly mean the end of the war. Maybe this would be all there was that they would have to go through . . .

The bells rang from the church spires on Sunday, and the townspeople spoke proudly about how they seemed to sound brighter, clearer, than they ever had during the reign of the Fascists; and all the shops were open. People went back and forth on bicycles and in little cars. Children played in the rubble and dust and in the ponds of water that formed from the few squalls of rain that came in off the sea. It was a coastal city and already there was work on the damages of the invasion.

And the invading force, Marson's portion of it anyway, was stationary, nothing to do but clean and drill and wait. Mario took to coming into the bivouac to see Marson. Merchants, clergy, others were allowed past the perimeter as well. Mario would come in with bottles of wine under his shirt. "For my friend with the hole in his smile," he said.

NINE

On the side of the mountain in the rain, Marson and Asch were awake. Marson decided to let this pause go on a little, for the trembling in his own legs, and the stabbing that he felt with every step. Joyner slept on, though he fidgeted some, his legs jerking. Now and then little plaintive sounds came from him. The old man lay as still as any corpse, cloak pulled half over his head. Marson had also given him his blanket roll. The rock shelter smelled like a basement. There was also the redolence of rotting leaves, mixed with the stale damp odors of the men.

"I don't wanna sleep," Asch said, low. "Ever again. Every time now I go to the fucking desert and see that burning tank. Christ. You figure."

"You've got *me* seeing it," Marson said.

"I don't think I'm afraid of dying. I'm afraid of suffering."

Marson said nothing.

"That woman just stopped. Like that. Dead before she hit the ground. Out like a light. It's worse than the tank, and I'm scared I'll start dreaming that."

"Asch, can we talk about something else?"

"Sure. You wanna plan next year's prom?"

Marson let this go. He shivered and felt once more as if he would retch.

"You believe in God?" Asch said.

"Yes."

"I think it's all one thing. I mean one reason for all of it — the religion and the philosophy and all of the rest."

"Do you mean that all religions are true?"

"They're all there for the same true reason, yeah. It's all trying to explain the one thing. Why we have to die. It's all a puny attempt to deal with that fact."

"Well," Marson said. "That's how *you* see it."

"Listen to the prayers — they're all about save us from it, from the big bad dark. Every single religion. I think they all exist not necessarily because there's a God but because there's death. They're all trying to explain that away somehow."

"Every human civilization or social group, every tribe, believes in a God."

"Yeah?"

"I guess we need a God."

"That's it, then? And you're religious. It's just a practical decision?"

"Yeah," Marson said. And then nodded. "Yeah, sure, why not? Practical."

"Shit, just because you *need* it?"

"But look where that leads. Name one thing human beings need that doesn't exist. We need food, there's food. We need air, air. We need love, there's love. We need hope, there's hope."

"Okay, what about money?"

"You're gonna tell me there's no such thing as money?"

Asch pondered this.

"And there's also how you live your life," Marson told him. "What you do while you're here."

"You mean like shooting a helpless woman in cold blood?"

Marson was silent.

"Yeah," Asch said. "And all this — all this — this destruction — that's a response to it, too. And it's just gonna go on forever or until they find some way to kill everybody."

"Like I've been saying, Asch — you are the most morbid son of a bitch I know."

" 'The truth will set you free.' "

"I don't want to talk about this," Marson said. "You think all this hasn't occurred to

68

me? You think I haven't had these thoughts exactly? I don't want to talk about it or think it or hear it said, either. It doesn't do anybody any good. Not now. Not in this mess."

"Fuck," Asch said. "I'm just — talking."

"I agree with you about that — that business back down the road, too," said Marson after another pause. "But we've gotta get through this night, too. Right? What good does it do to argue with Joyner about it?"

"I don't know. He's so sure everything's a joke on everybody else."

Marson drank from his canteen and then held it out to catch the rain.

"I got enough bad imagery in my head to last two lifetimes," Asch said. "I don't know how I'm gonna get rid of it all."

In his mind, Marson saw the eyes of the man he had shot, the curved smudged calves of the woman's legs jutting from the wet grass.

"I don't think any damn church is gonna help me," Asch said. "I wish like hell it could. I'd be in the front row."

"Act as if you have faith, and faith will be granted."

"Is that so. You believe that."

Marson remembered being at a mass in Palermo. The company chaplain, a balding priest named Prentice, said the words *Hoc est enim corpus meum* and held the host up, and Marson believed he could feel the strength flowing into him from the words and what they signified. The church was a bombed-out building, some sort of community hall, and when the mass was over two soldiers walked in casually, talking about the cold water of the beach, and with the practiced gestures of old habit removed the crucifix and the tabernacle, wheeling them aside like so much furniture. Marson, who had remained behind to pray, saw this and was appalled. For a long time the fact of it disturbed him and broke through the flow of his thinking. It gave him a disagreeable sense of being privy to a sordid secret. All his young life, he had been adept at concentrating his attention, diverting himself from unwanted thoughts.

"My grandfather," Asch said. "The one who fought for the Kaiser. He was in the war to end all wars, I believe they, uh, called it. Yeah — that was it. Well, I've read the histories and the philosophies, too. This is not ideas we're fighting about, here. No matter what anybody says. They don't like Jews at home either. Or the blacks. The Nazis' *ideas* don't really mean shit. It's all just — better weapons. The ideas are just excuses. Just — we're getting better and better at killing. That's what it *is*. We've got the mechanisms for wider and more efficient killing. It's got nothing to do with ideas."

"You don't really believe that," Marson said.

"If it wasn't the Krauts it'd be somebody else. And it ain't ever gonna end, either. Not until there's nobody left to kill. Between 1600 and 1865 you know how many years of collective peace there were? Years where nobody was killing anybody in armies anywhere in the world? Eleven. Eleven little years, bud. Think of it."

"Where'd you get that statistic. You made that up."

"I made a study. It's true. And try counting up the years of peace since then." Asch stared out at the raining dark.

"Christ," Marson said. He saw in his mind the dead woman's legs jutting out of the drenched grass.

"I guess we have to go to battalion headquarters first," Asch said. "Don't we?"

"There's the chain of command."

"You wanna talk to *Glick* about it?"

"I guess we go to the captain. An officer anyway. Some officer."

A little later, Asch said, "You think it'll ever stop raining?"

71

"No."

"I wish we were back in Palermo."

"I wish I was back in Washington, D.C."

"You think Glick would shoot somebody to keep'm from reporting him?"

"Hey — I said I wish I was back in Washington, D.C.," Marson told him. "Try and get some sleep, why don't you."

"Can't sleep. I close my eyes and drift and it's carnival time with the burning tank." Scrunching down against the base of the rock, Asch looked like a puffy little boy in clothes that were too big for him.

They were quiet for a few minutes, and now Marson saw that the other man had indeed drifted off.

TEN

The gap in the corporal's teeth had been caused by getting hit with a baseball when he was about fifteen years old — Mario's age. The ball knocked the one tooth out, and the others grew toward the space, nearly closing it. He explained this to Mario, who wanted to talk about baseball from then on, being, as he said, a New York Yankees fan. No one in the world loved the Yankees like Mario, according to Mario, but among players he had a special affection for the New York Giants player Mel Ott, who lifted his leg when he swung at the ball and still hit home runs. "I know he has failed to hit as many home runs as Ruth, that is true, but Ruth don't have the difficulty of having to lift his leg when he swings at the ball. Is this not right?"

"That's right," Marson said, amused. "You know more about this than a lot of Americans."

"I am a fan. I know from the dictionaries that the first three letters from the word *fanatic* are *fan*."

Marson laughed. "Hell, kid, *I* didn't realize that one."

The boy stuck his chest out. "I love all things from your country."

"Well, I'm impressed. All this from one summer."

"I have followed it in the papers, signore."

"I see that."

Mario shrugged and half smiled, with his missing tooth. "Anyway, I never saw Ruth."

"He was gone by the time you got there."

"Oh, far gone, *sì*. The Chicago team."

"That's right."

"But of his former self, *una voce*. A rumor, yes?"

Marson smiled. "Yes."

"Still, people told me stories about this man so big in everything he did, this *personaggio leggendario*, a fable already."

"A man with a big potbelly from excess," Marson said, making a phantom circle around his middle with his arms.

"Excess," said Mario. "Fat?"

Marson explained about too much of everything.

"Oh," the boy said. "Like my gap-toothed friend and his friend Asch."

74

Marson grinned. "All right. Sure. Though not as much."

"Little bit," Mario said. "Not as much. Yes."

"Yes. And he — Ruth — he had these spindly little legs, and he could drink twenty bottles of beer and down sixteen hot dogs and still go to the ballpark and hit three home runs in a single game."

"And he also built the ballpark."

"Figuratively," Marson said.

"What is that: *figuratively?*"

"Like a picture. Making a point. He didn't actually build the stadium."

Mario thought a moment. The look of concentration on his face made him wholly beautiful. Marson felt a thrill of affection for him. He had a moment of hoping that if he lived to have sons, all of them would be as inquisitive and expressive and sharp as this dark charming boy, with his habit of reading the English news and listening to radio not to lose the language he had learned in one happy summer in New York.

"I only got to watch Gehrig, and the other one, DiMaggio," Mario said.

The corporal reached over and patted his shoulder. "You're a good man, Mario."

The boy was evidently thinking about having seen the great Gehrig and DiMaggio.

75

"Wondrous players but, you know, also right-handed."

"Well," said Marson. "Gehrig was left-handed."

"He was?"

"I'm sure of it."

"You say Gehrig *was*. He died, then?"

Marson nodded.

The boy frowned darkly, processing the information. He rubbed his lips with the long fingers of his left hand, then held them up and looked at them, as if searching for some answer there, something in the lines of his own palm. "I believe I read that." He sighed. Then: "Yes, I believe I did."

"A great ballplayer," Marson said, wanting to change the subject.

"Well, Gehrig and Ruth and Ott, all left-handers, then. *Si?* And I am left-handed, too. I love left-handed people and I feel myself to be a brother to them all."

Marson did not tell the other, as he was sorely tempted to do — in that friendly rivalry between boys — that he had been a left-handed pitcher in the Washington Senators organization for almost two years. To do so would've meant having to talk about it, and he did not want to do that anymore, did not want to think about being home and playing baseball, since it dejected him so much and made him realize with such sorrow where he actually was.

Each morning he prayed for the strength to do what would be required, and every single minute he felt like curling up and crying. He kept all this deep inside and never showed any of it to anyone.

Time passed more slowly than he would ever have believed possible. He took to trying to trick his mind by not looking at the time, would do whatever there was to do, forgetting his watch, believing that not to be aware of it could make the passage of the hours seem quicker. He was doing this, working at it one morning, sweeping refuse from the long platform where a temporary mess had been set up. He had seen that it was five minutes past seven in the morning, and he kept his eyes averted, working on, losing himself in the rote motion, imagining what everyone was doing in the late night of back home, the nightclub hour, the hour of all the talk and the music, when the pretty photographers came around and snapped the photos of everyone and offered the pictures for sale, and the cigarette girls walked up and down with their little strapped-on trays and all the choices; it was the hour when people were getting out of movie houses and yawning in the street, waiting for a taxi to take them to some quiet place for coffee or a cocktail. Five minutes past seven o'clock in the morning in Sicily, and Marson imagined it all, back home, a reverie he had fallen into, and when he realized it and shut it off, he felt certain that at least the hour of his dreaming must have gone by. He checked the time again: nine minutes past seven.

Four minutes.

He almost howled from the frustrated rage that came over him. He took the watch off and threw it over the wooden fence that bordered the makeshift mess hall where he was. But then he went looking for it that afternoon with the feeling of trying to find a precious part of life and with the fear of having lost it forever. When he found it, he stood holding it in the shadow of a blasted tree and wept, not even looking around himself to be sure he was alone. He packed it away among his things. And a little later he sent it home, with a note asking his brother to keep it for him.

The gap between his teeth gave him a tough, determined look, whereas Mario, with his missing tooth, just looked simple-minded. But Mario was nothing of the kind. He was quite proud about the wine and claimed that he knew every hiding place the

Italians had used to keep the best of it from the Germans. Mario said the Italians — the Sicilians, anyway — hated the Germans more than the Americans or Brits, as he called the English, ever could. The Germans were not slow, he said, but their beliefs made them stupid. Because they believed as they did, they were prevented from receiving certain insights and perceptions, such as the truth that the people of an ancient town like Palermo would have the courage and the intelligence to hide the good wine. It was happening all over Italy, Mario said with pride. The Germans had been fooled into thinking that Italian wine generally was grossly overrated. But Mario would provide Robert Marson (he pronounced it "Marsone") with the good stuff.

They were all awaiting orders. The rumors kept flying that the Germans were on the run, and nobody was supposed to talk about any of it. There was a report that General Patton had heard two troops speculating about what Italian coastal city would be the site of the invasion and that he'd had them arrested and sought to have them both shot for treason. General Eisenhower, the story went, had prevented it. Patton got reassigned north, and that fed the rumor that it was true.

All you could do when it came to talk, then, was talk about home. Because home, really, meant everything else, everything that wasn't the war: women, buddies, sports, jokes, music, children, food, drinks, cars, parents, school, houses. Home. But it hurt to talk about home. Marson dreamed of Helen. He put his hands on either side of her lovely face and kissed her, crying. And woke, crying. He wiped his eyes in the dark, buried his face in the pillow, and suffered in hiding.

The weather cooled slightly toward the middle of August and the sky was clear and blue over the darker blue sea in the mornings. The days dragged on. It got easier and easier to believe that nothing would change.

In the evenings, Mario would come around, and Robert Marson would call to him. "Paisan," he would say. "Come play poker with us."

"*Sì*," Mario would answer. "You will all lose money." It was like a ritual speech. They expected the exchange, and they never seemed to notice that it was the same, every time. Mario had told them that he had been taught to play by his father long before the summer he spent in New York. His father had learned the game from the Europeans who used to visit the island before Musso-lini and the war and the Germans, back when this, like much of Italy, was a place for wealthy people to come and spend money. "You will owe me your houses," Mario would say, cheerfully. "You will all pay." For Marson, it brought to mind something he had read once, how Caesar had played some card game with his cap-tors, the Gauls, saying repeatedly and jovially how he would escape and come back and hang them all, and how he had indeed escaped and then come back — and kept his word. And Caesar had been an Italian. And the killing had been going on unabated all the centuries. Marson had the thought and considered its uselessness. He did not finally care about any of it, but looked down at his own hands holding cards and wanted them never to be dead, wanted everything in the world to be different and better.

Mario was a bad, inattentive, helplessly social poker player, who wanted to chatter and tell stories and hear stories and seemed not to care a whit about the money, and often he quickly lost what little he had — no one knew where he got it to begin with — and Marson would stake him, for the wine.

"Mario," Marson would say after the first

few hands. "Vino."

"Chianti, Mar-sone?"

"Montepulciano, this time."

"Serious."

That was the boy's word, and Marson knew how he meant it, without having to think about it. It was something only between the two of them, a form of respect. A man was serious who asked for good wine and who knew how to appreciate it.

Marson had knowledge about wine because his father had taught him. The old man, Charles, also brewed his own beer, and in the summer of 1929, when Marson was twelve, the workmen building houses in Piqua, Ohio, where the family then lived, would come to the door of the house and say to his mother, "Mrs. Marson, do you think we could have a little of Charles's cold home brew?" Everyone in that town knew Charles, because of the brew and because of what he knew about wine. The German whites, the French clarets, and burgundy. But the old man loved Italian and Spanish wine best. Chianti, and Grenache. And cold, cold beer. When Marson turned fifteen, his father gave him a frosted glass of lager. "You can have a whole life of pleasure with this stuff if you learn to *taste* it rather than look for any strength or comfort in it."

At twenty-six, the young man was familiar with all the available pleasures of good drinking. "Mario," he would say. "Vino. Valpolicella this time."

"Serious," Mario would say.

Marson and Asch would follow him to the edge of the perimeter and watch him go on up the long prospect of the shadowed narrow alley, leading away from the water. The boy would dissolve in distance, and the dark, and they would go back to playing, the game lighted by a candle stuck down into a Chianti bottle, and in a little while Mario would return with the wine, three or four of the unlabeled bottles. It tasted always cool and dry, and they drank it from water glasses and jars, sitting in the flickering light and getting easy in the blood. Marson would lie down on his pallet those nights and, against all efforts not to, would think of Helen, seeing the little half-moon scar — the result of a fall when she was five — below the right side of her mouth, that widened when she smiled.

ELEVEN

Corporal Marson, the only one awake in the freezing darkness, considered that he would keep a watch over the others. Maybe the rain would lessen at last, and they could proceed without being drenched. Alone, he opened a tin of rations and tried to eat. His stomach wouldn't accept it. He moved off a few paces, into the downpour, and retched up what little he had swallowed.

He told himself that things had happened too fast for him to think. He replayed the scene in his mind — the shapes in the muddy straw, as if the two people were made out of it, emerging from it in a stream of epithets, the shots from the black Luger, Hopewell and Walberg falling, and his own shot, knocking the man over, the pale German with his bright red hair and his green eyes. It was all out of the realm of time in some way, and then time slowed while the Kraut died, and the woman kept shrieking, and Marson could not take his gaze away from the look of wonder in the dying man's eyes, until he heard the last shot, and turned to see the woman fall over, the legs coming up in that clownish inertia and thwacking back down in the mud. He should have walked over and challenged Glick about it then. The truth was that he had stood staring in sick amazement. He was still filled with that same feeling.

He saw Walberg and Hopewell as they had been that morning and in the hours of the day. He couldn't help himself. He saw Hopewell talking about Miami. The warm air coming in off the sea; the sweet nights with the sound of the waves. "Man, just try if you can and think about the music of the shoreline," he said, "those waves have been coming in like that for millions of years. Makes you feel small. Makes you see how little you are, how insignificant your problems are. Try if you can to think about that water, rolling in under the stars and under the sun over and over like that forever."

McCaig had said, "Try if you can to see how full of shit you are, Hopewell."

"It's true, though," said Hopewell. "I'm full of shit, all right, but that don't stop it all from being true. It's true."

And Walberg, talking about his father.

"My dad," he would begin. It was always a story involving the man's prowess. His wit. His escapades, some of which were rather unconvincingly exaggerated. "My dad set a blanket down and put food out for his first sophomore class, a picnic, you know, in the middle of the Lincoln Memorial. Right under Lincoln's statue." A look would come to his dark eyes, an anxious widening of them, as if he understood quite well that no one would believe him, and yet he was compelled to tell the story. Probably it was a story his father told. And it was clear that, for reasons of love, or pride, *he* believed it. Walberg. That boy, with his clumsy ways and his big feet and his soft chin that made him look always as if he were about to cry. Walberg never knew what hit him, and everything of him was gone now, all of it, the memory and the stories and the hope of being as funny and entertaining as the others — the desire to be a storyteller, like Marson — and the generations, too. Generations. His children, and their children. The thought went through Marson like an evil vapor.

Twenty-two years old. Walberg. His parents were probably not yet aware of what had happened to their just-grown boy. Hopewell's parents, too, were probably, like so many, oblivious to what was heading toward them across the awful curve of the world. Hopewell was only twenty. At that age, Marson was pitching a baseball in Charlotte, North Carolina.

He went back to the lee of the rock and nudged Asch awake.

"Christ, not yet," Asch said.

"Tell me," Marson demanded, "why you haven't reported it about the woman."

"I don't know. Leave me alone, let me rest."

"When I was twelve, I saw two guys in a fight. It was the first time I saw anything like it. The sound it made — fists hitting the faces. These two guys, teenagers. They danced and boxed, one coming forward and one backing away, and there was a thin line of blood around the one's mouth — the one who was coming on. They must've traveled a mile or more in that dance. And I followed them."

"Good for you," Asch said. "What the fuck are you telling me?"

"I was fascinated."

"Yeah?"

After another space, Asch said, "You're saying we were fascinated?"

"No. I don't know. I just thought of it — hell."

"I'll tell you," Asch said. "I couldn't believe it and then I could believe it. And it was *not* anything to do with politics or the liberation of Europe, you know?"

Joyner stirred and sat up. "Can you guys shut the fuck up?"

"We should move soon," Marson said.

But then they were all three very still, listening. Something was moving in the trees beyond the ledge. They got closer to the rock, waiting, trying to hear through the sound of the rain. Angelo sat up suddenly, and the sound beyond them stopped. They were all looking out into the pouring dark, and the old man wrung his bony hands and murmured something that sounded like praying. Perhaps five full minutes passed, in which no one moved or looked to one side or the other. The sound was there again, embedded in the incessant thrumming of the rain.

In the next moment, with a kind of haughty obliviousness, a deer walked slowly past where they were. It was a doe, and she stopped to look at them, only half curious, then went on, stepping neatly through the leaf and pine-needle slickness of the way down.

"She better not go down to the road. She'll be breakfast," Asch said.

They were all quiet again, a kind of aftershock from the alarm of something other than themselves moving in the dark. Marson offered Angelo some water from his canteen, and Angelo produced a little bottle of something that smelled of peppermint — it was schnapps. He drank from it and held the bottle toward Marson.

"*Per calore.* Hot your blood."

Marson took a sip. It burned all the way down and caused his gorge to rise yet again. Asch had gone back to dozing, and Joyner, too, seemed to be nodding off. But Joyner had seen the schnapps, and though he was a teetotaler he reached over for it.

Marson said, "This is schnapps, Joyner."

"I don't care. I'm fuck'n freezing." He took a pull of it. "Goddamn," he said, swallowing. "It tastes like candy." When he handed the bottle back, he said, "In a situation like what happened yesterday, everybody ought to keep his fuck'n mouth shut."

Marson made another try with the schnapps, and this time it went down smoothly. He gave the bottle back to Angelo, who put it under his cloak and then sat there nodding and muttering, hands tight on his knees.

"No matter what," Joyner said. "We're all guilty now because we didn't report it. We gotta just keep the fuck out of it."

The rain kept coming. Marson thought of home and then tried not to. He had never seen weather this extreme go on for this long.

Asch sat up and looked around. He had apparently been dreaming again. "God-damn it," he said through gritted teeth. The old man offered the bottle of schnapps to him and he took it, drank from it, then wiped his mouth and said, low, to Marson, "Where's Mario when we need him."

Marson got up and moved off again, and urinated into the cold running of the rain down the side of the mountain. Here was this humble need, that he had been answering his whole life, and standing there he felt as though he were something set down in the world from a profound distance, another species altogether.

TWELVE

He had met Helen when he was eighteen years old. They dated for six years before they were married, and during these nineteen months in the army, he had thought with regret about how he could have been a husband and father much sooner. In that other life he had used baseball as an excuse, a reason not to take on responsibility. He knew that now. He had always assumed he would one day have a family; he believed in that. He wanted to be in the world as his father was. But all of it was something he had imagined in a distance. He was in possession of a talent for throwing a baseball very fast. The ball jumped, moved when he threw it. He was very difficult to hit. And he did well on the farm team. There was talk of sending him up. It became easy to believe he would actually walk out on the perfect green expanse of a major-league ball field and pitch a game. He was that good.

And perhaps nothing else would have made his father more proud. But in the third year, a stubborn tendonitis developed in his throwing arm, and then Pearl Harbor happened, and the war was upon him.

His father had worked for the navy yard since '37, having brought the family to Washington after the failure of the farm equipment business in Ohio. He got the job thanks to Roosevelt's New Deal, and he was a Roosevelt Democrat. This was not an automatic thing with him: Charles Marson knew politics and kept up with all of it like some men follow sports. His own parents had come to America from Frankfurt, Germany, in 1893. He was Lutheran by birth, and he had made a pledge to a dying aunt, who knew of his interest in a young Irish Catholic girl named Marguerite, that he would never convert to Catholicism. He married Marguerite in 1916, with the promise that the children would be raised Catholic. He would not himself go to the church, but he would see that they did. Robert Marson's mother was from Irish immigrants, the Delanceys, all of whom had settled in the Ohio Valley in the middle of the nineteenth century. They had come for freedom — not from political or religious oppression but from hunger. Marguerite had the rare quality of being very devout while also being quite forbearing. She allowed differences between people, and when the workmen in the neighborhood asked for a bottle or two of her husband's home brew, she invariably provided it for them, like a woman in wartime feeding hungry soldiers — all of this while having never tasted any kind of alcoholic beverage in her life. And all of this before the Depression, and the war.

Her husband was tall, strong, blond, fierce eyed, direct, a man whose respect you wanted, and people usually did what he asked them to do. He had a way of talking in pronouncements at times. It was difficult for his children to believe he was not certain of the truth of every utterance. Marson knew his father's self-assurance had a cost: being the oldest, he had been privy to some of the doubts and worries, the hesitations, about the move to Washington. Charles had fought in the first war, in France. He had a shrapnel scar just below his elbow — a lozenge shape of lighter flesh — and on his left wrist and right cheekbone there were beaded lines where fragments of metal had grazed him. He was intensely patriotic, and sometimes his son felt this as an unexpressed — even unaware — form of compensation for the fact that he was of German blood.

Marson's last evening as a civilian was spent at his parents' home, where he and Helen had been living since the marriage. They all had a sad, quiet dinner, Robert, his brother Jack, who could not go to the war because he had asthma, Robert's young sister Mary, Helen, and his parents. Several times the dinner was interrupted by Marguerite's trips to her bedroom to cry quietly into her pillow — it was her way, had always been her habit when something hurt enough to bring tears. Helen sat weeping without trying to hide it, holding the ball of her belly where the baby was, and not eating, but with a cigarette smoldering in the ashtray by her plate. Jack smoked, too, and talked of how he wished he could come with Robert. He wanted to serve. Near the end of the meal, he got up from the table and went up to his room and was gone awhile, and Marson thought he, too, might be crying into his pillow. But he came back down, and he had with him the title of the car Marson had bought in the summer, a Ford sedan.

"What's this?" Marson said to him, only beginning to understand.

"I'll keep it clean as a whistle for you," Jack said. "And of course no one will drive it anywhere until you get back."

"What'd you do?"

"He paid it off," Marson's father said. "You own it outright."

Marson stood and embraced his younger brother, and then stepped back and shook his hand. "You didn't have to do that, Jack. But I'm so glad you did."

"I thought you would be," Jack said, as if he were joking, but his eyes welled up. Marson put his arms around him again.

When it was time to go, he hugged Mary and then his mother, and he allowed her to hold his face in her nervous, thin, cool hands, to look into his eyes that last time. Then he stood holding Helen Louise for a little while, with one hand resting on her abdomen, the lightest touch. His father walked with him out to the end of the sidewalk, where a taxi waited to take him to the train station. Jack and the women and the little girl waited on the porch, Marguerite with a stricken look on her face — but she was not crying now, would not cry — and Helen with her hands folded over the baby in her belly, fingers knotted so that the knuckles showed white. She, too, was managing not to cry, now. Mary was gripping the porch rail, smiling at him through her own complicated feelings. She was only eight, and all this leave-taking, and the talk of the war and distant places, was hard for her to understand. Marson waved at them and blew a kiss. It was a warm twilight, and the stars were beginning to show above the tree line behind the house. It came to him that he had taken this scene, this street, these people, for granted, had simply accepted all of it, and them, as his world. He had a thought: *this is the surround.* Just the word, *surround,* in that sentence, seemed freighted with new meaning. It could not be spelled any other way, was not the word *surroundings.* It was a different word. It was his life itself, containing his home, these parked cars, this house, this sky. Twelve thirty-six Kearney Street, Washington, D.C. *The surround.*

It caught his breath.

His father wanted to have a word with him. The others were shapes now in his peripheral vision.

"I have two things to say to you," Charles said, shaking hands with him.

The younger man held the grip, looking directly back into the somber blue eyes, because he knew it was expected of him. They were two men, standing face-to-face. It meant everything to Marson to be standing there with his father in that way, grown, with a wife of his own and a baby on the way. It caused a little catch in his throat when he tried to speak, so he cleared his throat and kept silent. His father dropped his hand and then put the end of his right index finger on the son's chest, a light but insistent touch.

"Do your duty," he said, and, surprisingly, *his* voice broke. He took a breath, then stepped back. "And write to your mother."

"Yes, sir," Marson told him.

Charles took him suddenly by the shoulders, but then let go.

"Remember."

"I will, sir."

"Don't miss the train."

"No, sir."

The old man's eyes were brimming. He had come from Germany. *His* father never spoke a word of English. Marson looked at the porch, Helen's anguished face, his mother's, Jack's, and Mary's, and he raised his hand to wave, then took one more glance at the street, and his father, and with a kind of wrenching shoved his duffel bag into the backseat of the cab and got in.

"Train station?" the cabbie said.

Marson couldn't talk. Through the blur of tears, he saw the cabbie take one look at him in the rearview mirror. The cabbie

97

leaned slightly toward the passenger window and spoke to the boy's father. "I've got a son heading out tomorrow," he said.

Marson's father held up one hand to acknowledge it. Then he stood close to Marson's window. "Come home in one piece. We'll all be praying."

"I will, too."

The cab pulled away, and Marson watched his father's shape grow smaller in the fading light of the street.

Thirteen

On the cold hillside — or mountain — near Cassino, Corporal Marson let the freezing hour pass, dreaming of home. His life there now seemed a hundred years ago. Or it was worse than that: sometimes, now, in the nights, it felt like something he must have imagined. It no longer carried with it the weight of memory but was marbled with the insubstantial feeling of imagination when the faculty for imagining is sketchy or false. He could not really believe it happened, any of it.

And, here, in the middle of a war, in the stupid prodigality of killing all around him, he had been witness to a murder.

He saw Joyner stir and look up. Joyner emitted a soft whimper and then began trying to move his fingers. Joyner turned to Asch, who made a sound like talk, a word that was indistinguishable. "Shut up, Asch," he said. Then he looked at Marson. "It's not a hill. We can't find out anything climbing this fucker."

Asch sat up and put his hands to his face. "I say we go back. That's my vote."

"Shouldn't we go back?" Joyner said to Angelo, who did not know he had been spoken to. "Hey, Mussolini or whatever the fuck your name is."

At the mention of the name, Angelo turned to him. *"Come?"*

"His name's Angelo," the corporal said. "He's our guide. He knows the paths up this hill. You remember me, I'm the one with the stripes."

"Yeah, well ask him if this is a mountain."

"Montagna, sì."

"See?" Joyner said.

"Anytime you want to check out, Joyner — you just let me know."

"But, man," Asch said. "I don't think we were supposed to climb a mountain."

Corporal Marson looked at Angelo and made a gesture of questioning.

"Sì," said the old man. "Speaka the English. *Poco.*"

"Well, praise Jesus and pass the fuck'n ammunition," Joyner said.

"If we don't do anything," Asch said suddenly, "we're as guilty as Glick is."

"No," said Joyner. "She's guilty as who

she was with and she paid for it, too. Maybe you didn't notice that they *shot* two of us."

"*He* shot. She didn't do anything but yell. And die."

"Both of you shut up," Marson said. "There's nothing we can do about it now."

"Just quit talking about it," said Joyner to Asch. "It's getting on my nerves." He was scratching his arm again. "We were all in shock. Forget it, will you?"

"The longer we wait the worse it's going to be."

"You got a radio?" Marson asked him. "Do you?"

Asch merely stared back at him.

"We're going to complete this mission. Got it?"

The old man had a coughing fit, spat into his hands, and then put his hands down in the snow. It felt very strange having him there, and it was difficult to believe that he did not understand everything in their talk.

"Move out," Marson said. He touched the old man on his shoulder and felt bone. For some reason, it got the nausea roiling in him again. The old man sat up and hugged his own skinny knees in the burlap trousers. A few more moments passed while they packed the blankets and gear, and Marson watched Angelo wrap himself in his canvas-like cloak. He thought of his father and wondered if Angelo had many children or grandchildren, a wife who was alive.

An instant passed in which he saw himself trying to tell them at home about the death of the woman.

He shook his head, as if to dislodge something in his helmet. The old Italian man looked at him with a question in his eyes. But no one spoke. They were all about to leave the rock. But then they stopped, each realizing in the same instant that the world had grown hugely, unnaturally quiet. The stillness was startling and appalling. Looking at the dim shapes of one another in that tight little space, it came to them that the rain had stopped.

Joyner held out one hand, brought it back, but then seemed doubtful and put it out again. "Well goodness fuck'n gracious," he said. "Isn't that the sweetest little mothafuck'n thing. You know what it's fuck'n doing now? It's fuck'n snowing."

This seemed to stop them all. Asch gave forth a sound like a gasp and then took his helmet off and looked down into it, as if searching for some secret he had hidden there. He put it back on and sighed. "I think I've got frostbite already in my feet."

Marson remembered the blister on his

right heel. He stood. "Let's go."

They moved off the ledge, away from the shelter of the rock, and began to climb again, the old man leading the way. His motions seemed a little stiff now, a little slower. The snow was covering everything quickly, the ground turning white at their feet, and ahead of them, too. It was gathering thickly on the branches of the trees and on every crease in the ground, softening all the crevices and dips and the little ridges and wrinkles of the earth, covering the dead leaves and the windfall as if to hide them all away in whiteness. Walking was becoming even more difficult. The tracks they made were black, and when they slipped there were swaths cut in the whiteness, like wounds. The flakes were very heavy with moisture, dropping with a kind of silent splash, but the flakes themselves did not melt when they hit. They adhered to the surface and were added to, second by second, an impossibly rapid accumulation, and the ground kept getting steeper. Twice the men had to wait while one or the other of them collected himself after a fall — first it was Asch again, and then Marson, who felt in the first loss of footing, as he started down, that he would tumble all the way to the road below. But he caught himself at last, and climbed back toward the others. Joyner gave him the butt end of his carbine and helped pull him up. The old man watched them from the shadow of the floppy canvas hood. He was a dark shape in the whiteness. They all looked like shadows.

Marson's foot had grown progressively even more painful, the pain traveling from his heel to the side of the foot, and now he was experiencing shooting pains all the way to his hip. He called for another pause, and they gathered, a dark knot of shades, amid the black trunks and the outcroppings of rock, huddling together against the cold. They looked around them.

"I think we should go back," Joyner said suddenly, scratching his arm again.

No one answered him.

Marson waved the old man on. And they began climbing once more.

"This is shit," Joyner said. His voice carried in the silence of the snowfall.

Marson ignored him.

They went on without speaking, and their huffing and breathing seemed to grow louder. The snow gathered so quickly, thickening, and now they had to lift their feet out of it and put them back down again, climbing, and the resistance of the gathered snow became another impediment.

Finally they reached another place where the slope leveled slightly, the brow of a crest, like a landing on a staircase, and this led into a clearing. The trees opened out and fanned to the left and right. The four men walked a little ways into the opening. It was a meadow. They could see the sky here, or something of the sky, a screen of the snowfall with the suggestion of moonlight behind it. Marson reflected that it was light, a kind of light. The snowfield was such a change from the trees, the crowded feeling of the trunks surrounding them as they climbed. They spread out and moved slowly into the clearing. The snow was pristine. There were no tracks and no hollows in it, no sign that anyone had walked here. They stopped again about fifty yards in. The old man fell on a hidden stone, startling the others, and they watched as he quickly tried to rise. The corporal helped him and felt the shivering in his frame. The old man was soaked, and the snow covered his head and shoulders. Marson unfurled his blanket and put it over him.

"It's a fucking blizzard," Joyner said. "We're lost."

"I'll tell you when we're lost," Marson said. But he did not believe himself.

"We could've wandered anywhere in this

shit," Joyner told him. "We could be three miles back down the fuck'n road and you know it."

"Three miles *above* the road, I know that," Asch said. He sat down — he seemed partially to collapse — in the snow.

"How much farther?" Marson asked the old man, who stood there shivering, holding the blanket tight around himself.

"*Capisco. Non lontano.* No far. *Ora è vicino.* Near. Near."

"The son of a bitch is lying," Joyner said, scratching.

Asch had lain back on his pack in the snow. "Shut up, Joyner," he said.

"Quiet," said Marson. "We'll take a break here, and then we'll go on."

"We're just gonna stay here until the fuck'n snow covers us."

No one said anything for a moment. And then they were down, facing out from one another, trying to peer into the trees. A sound had come from somewhere, a snapping of something, a branch falling, heavy with the snow — or a footfall. It made them all realize how exposed they were.

"Move," Corporal Marson said, "that way." They headed into the nearest trees, trying to keep low, though this was undoable because the snow impeded every step.

106

They kept having to lift their feet out of it, and it held them, made their flight a strangely farcical lurching and faltering, a ridiculous clownish rush. Asch even laughed, once, high and soprano sounding in the echoless silence, and Marson told him to shut up. The corporal's blistered and inflamed foot stabbed him with each lumbering step. But they all got to the trees and ranged themselves among the trunks, looking out at the blank face of the clearing with their tracks in it, going off in the dark.

After a long interval of waiting and listening, Joyner muttered, "There's nobody else on this fucker but us."

"You want to walk out into that clearing?" Asch said. "You go right ahead."

"I want to turn around and go back down, remember?"

"Well, we can't stay here."

The snow flew at them sideways now, the wind having picked up, blowing across the open space.

"You guys are Christians," Asch said. "You believe in an angry God who's interested in payback. Right? 'Vengeance is mine' — all that. Well, we're gonna pay for yesterday. I think we might be paying for it now."

"You're so full of shit," Joyner said. "Let go of it, will you? It's our religion so we're the ones who'll go to hell, not you."

"I'm not even going to answer *that*," Asch said. "Jesus, Joyner. The way your mind works."

"It's stupid to argue about it *here*," Marson said.

"I can't get the image of her legs out of my head."

Marson almost turned to Asch to say he had the same unwanted picture in his own mind. But the knowledge of it frightened him. He had again the obliterating sense that everything of his memory, everything of his knowledge and his dreams and the hopes and aspirations of his lived life, was in a kind of gray, lifeless suspension. Even the wish to be generous and to seek the good opinion of others. It was all elsewhere.

But he could not think about that now, could not let himself give it room in his mind. There was no place for it there, but only for getting through these hours of the cold and the rising wind.

Joyner and Asch were waiting for him to say something.

He looked out at the snowfield, then at his compass. He took the scope out of his web belt and panned the field slowly. He could see only the snow inscribing the shape of the wind. "We're gonna go until we can see what's beyond this," he said. "And we're gonna keep to the trees and go around." He took the old man by the elbow. "*Capeesh? Around?* You know the way?"

The old man nodded, gesturing toward the tree line. "*Si.* Around."

FOURTEEN

They kept as much as possible to the trees, with the dusting of snow limning the trunks on one side, the side where the wind was coming, raising a blinding cloud and stinging their faces. Marson's foot was now burning deep and was strangely numb at the same time. It seemed that the flesh around the abrasion, leading down into the toes, was dead. And the snow made each step a crucible, an agony. He kept trying to offer up the pain, but his concentration was breaking down. The old man's rope-soled shoes were packed with the snow, and he was shaking so visibly that again it became necessary to stop. Marson made the others gather close to him, to try warming him. The corporal's blanket was stiff with freezing, adhering to the old man's frame.

"Morirò di freddo," Angelo said, shivering.

"We don't understand you," Joyner said. "Fucking stupid —"

110

"Shut up," Marson told him.

"*Morirò*. Die. Wintry!"

"Yeah," said Joyner. "All of us."

"We're gonna have to build a fire," said Marson. "Look for a place away from the field."

"Shit. You think that's safe to do?"

They all waited, facing into the clearing on their left, as if listening for anything like another human presence in the acres of white before them, the crowding trunks behind. There wasn't anything but the sweeping flakes and the wind.

"I don't know," Asch said. "If anybody else is around they're building a fire, too, or they're gonna die."

Once more, they waited.

"Let's just stay awake and alert," Marson said at last, and led them deeper into the trees. They came to a hollow of sorts, a dip in the ground, in the lee of another stone outcropping. Asch and Joyner went off to forage for kindling, and the other two dug out a place just under the curve of the rock. It was difficult to tell which way they had gone now, how far from the other side of the mountain. It was even possible that they had retraced some ground, heading back down toward the road. The snow could've hidden their own tracks from them. According to the compass, they had been moving steadily east.

But the most important thing now was getting out of the wind.

Joyner and Asch were two ghost-dark shapes in the falling curtain of flakes, the wide whiteness out of which the snow-lined trunks of the trees rose. Their squabbling carried back, even in the face of the storm. Marson and Angelo sat against each other side by side, in the lee of the rock. The snow had turned to sleet, mixed now with more freezing rain. They huddled under the declivity, just beyond the reach of the worst of it, and watched Joyner and Asch come stumbling back, their arms full of the windfall for which they had had to dig. It took a while to build the fire, but when it was going, they hunched close, feeling the warmth.

It felt like the first warmth of the world.

Marson watched the ashes and embers rise into the snowing sky and felt them as an announcement of their position. But the crackling of the fire and the groaning of the branches above them were the only sounds now. Clods of snow shook loose from the tops of the trees and dropped like rags among the branches.

In the firelight, he looked at Angelo's face.

It was full of wrinkles and faintly dishonest looking — there was something about the way he kept glancing away. He had a long nose, and bony cheeks, and deep-socketed eyes that, in the flickering, suggested the skull beneath the flesh. There was a thin downturning of the mouth on either side, a permanent frown. On his forehead were two marks, upside down Vs, like little scars, and you thought of nails until you realized it was the way the wrinkles in his brow gathered, just under what would've been the hairline. When he opened his mouth to speak, you could see that the front teeth, upper and lower, were all he had, and the upper ones were in bad shape.

"Guide?" Marson said to him. "You know where we go? Guide? Still guide?"

The face did not register understanding.

"Shit," said Joyner.

Asch stared out into the dark, listening for movement.

"Angelo," Marson said, trying to remember what little Italian he had learned from Mario, those months ago — it felt like years — in Palermo. "*Perso?* Lost? Are we lost?"

"Near," the old man said, nodding in the direction of the field.

"He doesn't know where he is any more than we do," Joyner said. "He'd've said anything to save himself. He thought we were gonna shoot him. We're fucked."

"I wish you'd can it for good," Asch said.

"Yeah, let's just bury our heads in the snow. Operation Avalanche, remember? And here we are. Buried in the fuck'n snow." Operation Avalanche had been the name for the landing at Salerno.

"Both of you shut up," Marson told them. "Just shut *up!*"

"I say we head back down to the road. While we can still find the road."

"Near," said Angelo.

"Yeah," Joyner said. "Near. Near what?"

"Non capisco."

"Yeah, no *capeesh.*"

"I'm ordering you," Corporal Marson said.

They put some more pieces of wood on the fire. The flames rose higher, and the heat grew momentarily more intense. Asch moved into the circle and put his hands close, and Joyner turned his weapon on the field, where the snow had begun to let up. Above them, an opening began in the clouds, a thinning of the curtain. Something of the moonlight shone through.

FIFTEEN

The difficulty between Marson and Joyner had begun in Palermo. Joyner had been too worried about regulations, and he did not like the use of wine. His people had been very concerned with temperance. None of them drank, not even beer. He'd had trouble with stomach ulcers when in high school, and his mother had had them her whole life. He played in the poker games, but he neither smoked nor drank, and Marson did both, as did Asch and the others. Joyner's fund of curses and obscenities seemed inconsistent with such attitudes, but he did not see the irony. The language he used in daily talk was exclusive of his beliefs about behaviors regarding alcohol and tobacco. Mario, attuned to every nuance between the soldiers, realized this and began looking for ways to needle Joyner with the wine. He would offer it to him every time he picked up the bottle to pour more for Marson or

Asch or one of the others. Joyner tried to ignore him, but you could see that it was getting to him.

"Oh, yes. Signor Joyner does not drink," Mario would say, as if he had to remember it all over, each time.

During the landing drills, when they were put together in the landing craft, and Joyner would spill a stream of his obscenities, Marson would repeat Mario's phrase exactly, with exactly Mario's faintly chiding tone.

They were both buck privates then. Raw, fearful, and antagonistic.

Marson's ability to tell stories was a source of aggravation to Joyner, who liked to think he was good at it. It seemed to others that Marson had led a more interesting life, and of course he was older. Marson's time in boot camp included episodes of wild stupidity by a big brutal boy from Texas, named Wagoner, who got drunk every day somehow and deserved everything that his stupidity brought him. Marson had told a story about how Wagoner, after being stripped of his rank because of a fight he had picked at a saloon on the perimeter of the base, came to Marson and asked what he should do about the darker place on his sleeve, where the one stripe used to be.

Marson, who had Wagoner's trust because he was a storyteller and because the stories commanded the attention of others, told him to go to the supply shack and get some stencil letters and print DISREGARD on the sleeves. Wagoner had done so and had walked around the camp that way, through most of an afternoon, until a sergeant finally noticed it and chewed him out for not being in uniform.

Marson went on: "The DI would scream at the guy, 'Damn it Wagoner, don't you know we're at war?' And Wagoner would say, 'You know it, Sergeant, and boy I sure hope we win.' He had a sweat of booze on him every single morning and I swear I don't know where he got his hands on it."

"You don't know where I get the wine," Mario said. "But I am never mean or dumb."

"You bring it back, Mario, my friend. This guy drank it all. He never gave anything to anyone except a black eye or a busted lip."

Mario liked the story about the stripe and the stencil so much that he had the word DISREGARD scrawled on the sleeves of his T-shirts, and he was always after Marson to tell more Wagoner stories. Wagoner being carried asleep in his bunk out of a barracks and onto the gravel walkway that ran down the center of the camp. Wagoner getting drunk on Aqua Velva and passing out in the chow line. Wagoner curling up with his blanket roll so he could sleep better while on guard duty during war games. That was what finally got him washed out of the service, unfit for duty.

"Unfit for duty," Joyner said. "Smell that one."

The word *washout* became a favorite expression of Mario's, and he took to calling Joyner that, whenever Joyner would turn down yet another offer of wine.

"More wine, Signor Joyner?"

"I'm not even gonna answer you."

"Ah, a washout, then," Mario would say. Clearly, he was Marson's friend. And when orders came down and they were all gearing up for what they knew would be an amphibious landing somewhere on the mainland, Joyner came to Marson and said, "Your Guinea pal has got something for you."

"Wish I could take it with me," Marson told him. "Call him Guinea again and I'll fix your smile for you permanently."

"You can try to," Joyner said.

They were standing in the middle of the camp, which was being dismantled. They stood very close, and neither of them moved for a few seconds.

"Maybe you should save your anger for the Jerries and the Wops," Joyner said.

"Oh, I'm not angry," said Marson. "I'm just definite."

"Well, let's see how definite you are in ten minutes."

All around them, men were putting things into duffel bags and packs. It was a little frantic. This would be an enormous transporting of men and supplies, and they were going to be in the middle of the war and they knew it. They knew that a lot of them would be dead soon. The pall of that knowledge colored everything and made the sunny breezes from the sea seem dimly wrong even as they also felt unbearably precious.

"Your boy has something for you," Joyner went on, "and I'm not talking about your fuck'n wine." He pointed up the row of tents being dismantled. There was Mario, with a small boy and a man. The man had his arm around Mario's shoulder. All three of them were being prevented from entering the bivouac. Marson walked over to them.

"Signor Mar-sone." Mario smiled brightly with his missing tooth. "This is my father. Giuseppe."

Giuseppe was squarely built, bulky through the shoulders, with muscular arms and big, rough-looking hands. His face was large featured — a wide nose and round, heavy-lidded eyes, and a black hairline that came to the middle of his forehead. He said something to Marson in Italian, glanced at Mario, and then back at Marson. *"Per favore,"* he said.

"I'm sorry," Marson told him. *"Non parlo italiano."*

"This is my father," Mario said. "He's embarrassed by his English, so he speaks Italian to you." He made a motion as if to present the little boy, pushing the boy's skinny shoulders so that he stepped forward. The boy was even darker than Mario, sullen seeming, with a little purple scar the shape of a fishhook above the left eye. "My father wishes you to take my brother with you to America," Mario said.

Marson looked at him, and then at the boy, who was staring at his own small hands folded in front.

"Per favore," said the man. *"Per favore."*

"I —" Marson began.

"I know you can't take two of us. And my brother has never seen America." A light shone in Mario's eyes — a kind of sorrowful humiliation, a regret, and something of

120

pride and anger, too. "You must take him for the wine, Signor Mar-sone."

"Wait. Lord. Look," Marson said. "You think we're —"

"Il Duce will not last," Mario said. "Italy will surrender. It is over. Will you do it?"

"But I'm not *going* to America." Marson felt anger and tried to suppress it. "I wish I was. Look, Mario, I'm probably going to be dead tomorrow. We're all probably going to be dead. We're not — we're headed to the mainland. The invasion. Tell your father. It's an invasion. We're not going home. We're going to the war."

The man said something else in Italian, then turned to Marson. "*La mia famiglia.* Family."

"I understand," said Marson. "My family's five thousand miles away."

The man stared.

"*Capisco,*" Marson said.

"*Sì. Come voi, amo la mia famiglia.*"

"Like you," Mario translated. "He loves his family." The look in his eyes was almost ferocious.

"I do understand," Marson said. "I wish I could help."

Mario muttered something in the other language to his father, who appeared confused for a moment, but then, quite slowly,

121

showed the resignation of a man used to things turning out badly. With a sorrowful nod of his head he took the little boy by the hand and turned with him.

"I sell the wine," Mario said. "To the others I sell it."

"Yes."

"You, because of the hole in your smile. I get you the best."

"I know. I wish I could do something more." Marson had twenty dollars of overseas scrip in his pocket. He reached in and brought it out, a ten and two fives. He handed Mario the ten and one of the fives.

The boy glared at him, but took it.

"It's all I've got." Marson offered him the other five.

"You are a friend," Mario said. "Serious." And he walked away.

Marson watched him go. There was confusion and noise all around him, planes going over, and men shouting back and forth about the hell they were all headed to. It sounded like a lot of boys excited about going to a football game, until you heard the controlled desperation in it.

Joyner had come partway to the end of the row of tents, and he stood waiting. "You see what your goddamn wine drinking got you," he said.

Later, on the troopship headed for Salerno, news came through on the radio that the Italians were out of the war. Mussolini had been deposed. Everyone celebrated, and Marson had the thought that the mainland might be the same as it had been at Palermo. For some reason this gave him a terrible pang of missing home, of some kind of waste. The feeling surprised and alarmed him, and he looked out at the rise and fall of the sea, its little churning whitecaps, and was amazed at his own mind. Joyner came up to him and said, "We might actually miss this fuck'n war." He smiled and patted Marson on the shoulder, turning to gaze at the sea and sky with him. Asch walked over and offered Marson a cigarette. "Lucky Strike," he said. "Good name for a cigarette."

"That actually smells good," said Joyner. "You guys make me wish I smoked."

"You want one?" Asch said.

"Hell, sure — why not?"

Asch lighted it for him. He drew on it and did not cough. He kept the smoke in for a long time. When he let go of it the cough came, and the other two pounded his back and helped him through it.

"How do you guys stand it?" Joyner said,

still coughing.

"You get used to it," Asch said. "Takes work. I've been practicing to get better at it most of my life." He drew on his own cigarette and blew the smoke. Joyner tried it again and coughed less this time.

"It hurts my pipes, though."

"Maybe you should go easy the first time," Marson told him.

"Naw, I'll finish it."

They watched him smoke. He was getting the hang of it. He looked at Marson. "How much scrip did you give Mario?"

"All I had."

"You're gonna wish you'd kept some of it when we get to the mainland."

"It's only money," Asch said.

"That's kind of an unusual thing —" Joyner stopped. "Yeah, right. It's only money. Fuck it."

Asch shook his head, but smiled. There were cheers going up all over the ship.

They smoked their cigarettes and then tossed the butts over the side. In the happy feeling of the day's news, Marson stood between them and put his arms across their shoulders. Looking out at the red sun going down over the slow, ponderous agitation of the Mediterranean, he forgot all the tensions and slights and irritations of the last few weeks and felt as if these two were, after all, the best friends a man could have.

Sixteen

Crouched close to the fire, in the woods beyond the snowfield, Corporal Marson thought of the futility of money, and then he was thinking of the futility of everything. He tried to pray, and the words went off from him, as if addressed to the wind and the silence all around. Joyner had opened a can of vegetable hash and was heating it in the flames. He wolfed it down, someone filling a little hole, tasting nothing.

The old man watched him and then, seeing Marson's quiet gaze, looked down.

"Food?" Marson said. *"Mangiare?"*

The old man shook his head and smiled thinly. Marson wondered what he might be like, sitting at a table with people around it, and wine, and a peaceful countryside out the windows of a room. A warm countryside. He imagined it, the green grass in the gold light of an evening's sinking sun. And then he moved closer to the fire, shuddering. Joyner had finished with his rations and he tossed the empty can off into the snow, like a grenade, the same motion of the arm.

"I could be a father right now," Asch said suddenly. "That seems like an insane thought to me."

"You better quit thinking so much," Joyner said to him, reaching under the sleeve of his field jacket and digging at his forearm.

Asch ignored him, still looking at Marson. "Can't we call it, and go back down?"

"Asch wants to go back as much as I do," Joyner said.

Marson turned to the old man. "Take us."

"Non capisco."

He gestured toward the clearing. "Near. Bring us near. We move near."

"Oh, *sì*."

He gathered his cloak about him and stood. The others followed suit. The wind had dropped now, and the last of the snow filtered down out of the opening sky. Corporal Marson saw a glitter in the farthest distance, just above the tree line. The North Star. It thrilled him. There were little places in the sky beyond the trees, where the clouds were parting, like the fingers of a giant hand, once clasped, now letting go.

They covered the smoldering fire with

snow and trudged on, keeping to the trees, going around the field, another path the old man knew. He moved with the alacrity he had exhibited in the first hour of the journey. On the far side, the ground dipped for a few yards and then rose sharply again, and again they were climbing. But it was just the cold now, and the snow that had already fallen. They saw no tracks, no signs of life anywhere, until they reached another clearing, a small white level span of ground, leading to another tree line and more of the steep climb. In that clearing, standing quite still, was a large buck deer, with a prodigious rack of antlers ranged above its head. It was looking right at them, white breast jutting from just below the neck, its breath showing in frosty vanishing plumes from its black muzzle. The eyes were black, blank, staring. Marson felt eerily as if it had been sent by the doe they had seen earlier, to evaluate what sort of threat they were to the forest. It turned, so slowly as to seem gradual, then stepped away, thin legs looking almost spindly, the massive tawny-black shape adorned by the high white tail, moving off. It came to a large windfall, the trunk of a fallen tree, and leapt over it with swift ease, as though its containment in gravity were only provisional.

"Jesus Christ," Asch said.

They watched it go up through the trees, in the next level of this mountain they were climbing.

"There's no end," said Joyner, sounding as though he had wept the words out.

They came to the ascending ground and began climbing again, following the old man. There were tree shadows now, and Marson realized that the moon was high, and it had cleared the clouds in the lower quadrant of the sky. A clear night. The air was colder than it had been all day. It stung his bronchial tubes, yet he drew it in, felt the purity of it, the new, dry, clear air.

They were climbing. It was rote again, their thighs burning, the ground treacherous and shifting beneath them. For a time, the men followed the tracks of the deer, going off up the incline, but then the tracks wound through the trunks of the trees and disappeared.

"I've gotta shit," Joyner said suddenly. "God*damn* it."

They stopped. He went a few feet into the moon shade and took care of it, cursing. Angelo made a sound under his breath. There was no telling if it was a word or merely a grunt.

"God*damn* it," Joyner said, off in the near

distance. The noise of what he was doing went off from him and carried over the stillness.

Asch made a little snorting sound, a muffled laugh. "He's louder than a tank."

"*Il suo culo congelerà,*" the old man said.

"*Congelerà.* What the hell is that?"

"*Freddo.* Ice. Freeze-uh." The old man made a motion of being cold, arms wrapped around himself.

"Freeze-uh his ass, right?" Asch laughed. "Ass?"

"*Culo. Sí.* Freeze-uh his ass."

"Freeze-uh his *culo,* that's right." He kept laughing.

Joyner took care of himself as best he could with fingers that had grown numb and paper from his pack that was damp and cold. He cursed and sputtered.

They went on a little and then stopped to wait for him. The wind had died down, and there were very few clouds now. Joyner had finished and commenced getting himself together again, still cursing. From this distance, he sounded like a complaining little boy. He trudged up to them without making eye contact.

"*Siamo arrivati,*" said the old man, gesturing at the steep rise ahead. "*Quello è il posto.* There. Over there."

Joyner cursed again and muttered. Marson didn't hear him, and then he did. "We must be in fuck'n Switzerland by now."

"*La Svizzera,*" the old man said.

"Yeah, you understood that, mother-fucker."

They kept climbing. The ground leveled again and they saw that it stretched out away from them; they saw trees that looked short, like a tight row of firs, until they realized that they were the tops of trees. They had reached the crest and started across it, hurrying without realizing it, the old man leading the way.

They had gone about twenty yards when they heard a shot. One report, from no direction they could pinpoint. They all dove into the snow, even the old man.

After a few seconds of waiting, Marson murmured, "Anybody hit?"

Silence.

"Joyner?"

"I'm here. Goddamn it."

"Me, too," said Asch.

The old man murmured, "*Madre di miseri-cordia . . .*"

"That was a shot," Asch said, low. "A pistol."

"Did you get a sense of where?" Marson asked him.

"Shit — over there?" Asch pointed to the trees on the far side of the hill.

"You're sure it was a shot and not a branch breaking."

"It was a shot. Christ."

"But it was far. It was a long way away."

"You sure of that?"

"You can't tell distance at this height," Joyner said.

"Sound carries farther the higher you go, doesn't it?" said Asch.

They were whispering, but the whispering itself carried. It made them all the more nervous about what might be out there on the other side of the hill.

"Keep down," Marson said. "And stay quiet. Get back to the trees."

The wind had picked up again, rising from the north, and it lifted the snow, as if the hill, this meadow, were in the wildest heart of weather, above the snow line. It was the wind of the tops of mountains.

"Climb the hill," Joyner said. "Fuck." His scratching now looked frantic, as though something were crawling on him under the sleeve of the field jacket. "Go right on up the brow of the fuck'n devil."

"One more word like that from you," Corporal Marson said, "and I swear I'll shoot you myself."

"Fuck you, okay? This old man's led us on a wild goose chase."

"Shut *up!*" Asch said. "Marson's in charge."

They were still whispering.

"Close," the old man told them.

"It's all shit. We don't even know what's going on down on the road. The fuck'n Jerries could've turned on them and we're in enemy territory now."

"Shut up," said Marson.

They were quiet again, listening.

"We were fucked the minute Glick shot the whore," Asch said suddenly.

"Oh, that's great, Asch. We're cursed. Christ."

"Madre di Dio . . ."

"Everybody shut up," said Marson. "That's an order!"

The wind came over them with more force, and it made a sound, moving through the trees. The high, bare branches clicked and groaned and cracked. They were still heavy with snow and ice.

"How long do we stay here?" Asch said, low.

"Let's go," said Marson. "We'll go around again. Keep to the trees."

For a while they moved with stealth, from tree to tree, pausing a little at each one to listen. There was only the wind.

At last they came to a long narrow swath of open ground, between two rows of trees, with drifts of the snow in it. It was two banks, really, and it looked like a riverbed, or a lane. They went along it, crouching low, toward a large black object, a rock or a hillock, you couldn't tell. It blocked the bed, and when the old man reached it he abruptly stopped and held one hand out, waving them down. They scrabbled into the snow-laden second growth and waited, watching him where he knelt, using it for cover. They could see now that it was the root system of a big fallen tree. They heard water trickling somewhere. The old man waved them forward, and Marson went over to him. Just on the other side of the tree trunk was a small stream. It amazed him that the water was not solid ice. But the ice was melting. Just beyond the melting were the smoldering remains of a fire, and, within a few feet, a dark elongated shape.

In the instant of understanding that the fire was the reason for the melting, Marson realized that he was looking at the body of a man, lying flat on his back, arms out-stretched, as if he had fallen backward and been left that way.

SEVENTEEN

It was a German soldier, from the markings on his uniform, an officer. He had no effects with him, or near him. His helmet was gone. His overcoat was missing. The pockets of his trousers had been turned inside out. In the middle of his forehead was the perfect round blackness of the hole the bullet that killed him had made. The snow under his head was stained, and much of the snow beyond where he had fallen was splattered and dark. It looked black in the moonlight. His eyes were black, too, and open wide.

"Goddamn, I wanna go down," Joyner said, scratching. "This is fucked. This is fucked, man."

"Why would they shoot their own guy?" Asch said.

No one answered. Marson told them to get down, and they did so, because the old man had got down. They waited. None of them could see beyond the slope of the corridor of snow between the rows of trees. The little embers of the fire were still warm. There were many tracks in the snow around it.

"They've left him," Marson said, low. "And they haven't tried to hide that they were here. So either they're running, or they don't know *we're* here."

"*Tedesco,*" said the old man, peering out from the tree roots.

They crouched lower, quickly, and looked out. But the old man was apparently only commenting on the body.

After a few tense moments of watching, Marson said, "Yes. *Tedesco.*"

"What the hell are you saying to him?" Joyner demanded.

"The word means 'German.' "

"Well talk English, for Christ's sake."

They held quite still. There had been another sound. But it was just the wind stirring in the branches again. Snow dropped from one of the treetops, like a collapsing roof, and broke among the lower branches.

"We didn't see any tracks getting here," Marson said.

"We made contact," said Joyner. "We can turn around and go back down this fuck'n thing."

136

"It's all fucked because of the whore," Asch said, low. He spoke evenly, but in the moonlight his face looked contorted with fright.

"I want you both to shut *up,*" Marson hissed at them.

"Tedesco," said the old man.

Marson turned to Asch. "How many men do you think? From the tracks."

Asch leaned up and looked at everything. "I don't know. Ten?" They were whispering.

"It's more than ten," said Joyner. "If you ask me it's a *lot* more."

"Do you think they knew we were coming?" Marson asked.

"What the fuck are you saying?"

"They don't know about us," Asch said. "Or they don't care about us."

"I don't think they know," said Marson.

After another pause, listening for sounds, he murmured, "We'll wait a little. Let them get a good head start if they're running. And we'll be ready and waiting if they're coming back."

"Jesus Christ," Joyner said. "Aw, Jesus. You think they'll come *back?*"

"Just keep your eyes open," Marson said.

The old man had hunkered down against the tree trunk, with his knees up and his lower face covered by the cloth of his hood.

It was so cold, here. From the moon shade, his old eyes seemed ghostly. He stared at Marson. *"Freddo mortale."*

"Cold," Marson said.

"Sì. Freddo."

"We stay here for a time. *Capeesh?"*

"Stay, *sì."*

Marson looked through the scope, panning slowly across the open space and along the line of treetops beyond. The trail of footprints led away from the little campsite, and the wind, even now, was covering many of them, blowing the snow like sand. It was stronger and more steady now.

"It blew like this in Africa," Asch said. "But it was sand. I'd rather have the sand."

They fell silent again, waiting and listening. It was hard to say how much time went by. Before them, the body of the dead German was being gradually effaced by the blowing snow. The wind had shifted, coming fast from the west. Marson kept looking at what was left of the dead man's hair, and how the wind disturbed strands of it. There wasn't much that was clearly distinguishable anymore, because the drifting from the wind in its new direction kept sweeping across the little campsite, covering the embers, the tracks, the folds of frozen cloth on the body, and the features of the face.

Had they just now stumbled upon him, they would not be able to say what army he came from.

Asch moved back into the trees and urinated. When he returned he came low, gasping. He looked at Marson with a pleading expression on his face. But he said nothing.

"Go ahead," Joyner told him. "Make your complaint. It's cold. You frosted your little dick."

"I'm going to report what happened," Asch said.

"Jesus. *That* again. Mr. Broken Record."

"I'm reporting it. That's all I'm saying. I'm not going to go the rest of my life carrying this."

"Hey, who made you the moral compass of the fuck'n Fifth Army."

"I said we'd talk about it when we get back down to the road," Marson said. "This isn't the time. I'll go with you when the time comes."

"You're both fucked," Joyner said.

Marson kept glancing at the old man, who appeared simply to be observing the others as a man gazes upon birds feeding and arguing on a shoreline.

"Like I said, you might've noticed that two of us got it when she fell out of that cart."

Asch said, "She didn't do the shooting. For all we know she was a refugee, a victim."

"She was a Nazi, man. They don't like Jews. That's your people, isn't it?"

"Hey, fuck you, Joyner. *You're* a Nazi."

Joyner started toward him, but Marson got between them and held his carbine up, so that the barrel end nearly touched Joyner's chin. "Not one more word, not one more inch — *nothing,* Joyner."

The other's eyes were full of defiance, but he crouched back down and kept digging at the place on his forearm, muttering something about the itch that wouldn't stop.

Marson turned to Asch, still holding the carbine up.

Asch said, "Otherwise, we're no different than *they* are."

"Gotta have the last word," said Joyner. "Take it away, asshole."

"Close," said the old man.

"Sure," Marson said. "Near."

But they remained where they were, looking out at the snow corridor between the trees, the body lying there with the snow drifting over it.

EIGHTEEN

The wind glittered with snow, and the cold moon rose higher. It was sharper and brighter at the height of the sky. Corporal Marson thought of the stars as ice crystals. The trees made complicated striations of shadow, and the effect was like a ghostly daylight. Nothing moved before them. There was no sound anywhere but the wind. Marson watched Joyner where he crouched in the lee of the tree trunk with his carbine across his thighs, scratching the place on his forearm. The corporal believed now that the itch, as much as anything else, defined him.

At Palermo, when he first began to talk about the skin problem, there was no swelling or rash, no marks, no discoloration, just the itch. It had first come up when they were playing poker, and everybody but Joyner was drinking Mario's wine. Joyner would scratch the arm, and then scratch it again. He would look at it and shake his head, and then start once more, scraping and rubbing, looking at it and frowning. "Goddamn," he would say. And he would look along the arm, trying to find what it was on the skin that made it itch. He showed it to the others, and no one could see anything but the places where he had scored it, digging at it. He showed it once just as the itch began. The hair of the forearm stood up, as if some kind of static electricity were at work. "Look at that," Joyner said. "You guys tell me. That's the only thing it does, and then the itch. It's driving me out of my fuck'n mind." He grabbed the arm and scratched. "God*damn* it."

This kept up for days. He thought it might be sand flies, or chiggers, but the medic found no trace of any poison or bite. Joyner would keep scratching until it bled. And only after it bled would the itching stop. But then it would commence again a little farther up the arm or down toward the wrist, within an inch of the original site. The medic called it Irish skin.

"I'm nuts with it," Joyner said. "I want to cut the goddamn skin away. Peel it the fuck *off*."

That was way back at Palermo.

Now, he sat hunched over in the cold, huddled in the torn root system of the downed tree, and dug at himself, muttering low, glaring out at the moon-bright field, the top of the mountain. They were only a few hundred yards to a falling off, the descent on the other side. Marson watched him and worried.

"Put some snow on it," Asch said irritably. "Numb it."

"Fuck you."

They watched the field, the open ground. The old man began to cough. He choked up something and spit it out, then pulled snow over it, looking apologetically at Marson.

"How old do you think he is?" Asch wanted to know.

Marson said, "Angelo — how old?"

"Non capisco."

"*Età.* Your age." He knew the Italian word from Mario.

"Oh, *settantasette, anni.*"

Marson turned to Asch. "He's whatever that is."

"Seventy?" Asch said.

"*Sì.*" The old man shrugged.

"More than seventy." Asch gestured, raising one hand over the other.

"*Sì.*" The old man seemed confused.

"Goddamn," Asch said. "More than seventy. You're in some shape, ain't you."

"Good strong," Angelo said. *Molti bambini.*

"Bambini?"

"Sì." The old man held up both hands, fingers extended. He closed the hands and then opened one of them, extending four.

"That's fourteen," Asch said. "Damn."

"How many grandchildren?" Marson asked.

Angelo stared, smiling, and slowly lifted both hands again, all fingers extended, closed them, and then opened them again, and then closed them, and then held up the one hand with three fingers extended.

"God," Asch said. "Twenty-three?"

"That's too many Catholics," Joyner said. "Too many mackerel snappers." He laughed at his own joke. "How many of them are still alive."

This occasioned a silence. Marson did not know whether or not Angelo understood the question. His face was difficult to read. He looked at Joyner and seemed to be waiting for him to go on.

"Still alive," Joyner said. *"Capeesh?"*

"Sì," the old man said. "All."

"You're a lucky Fascist."

Angelo shook his head. "No."

144

"Not lucky?"

"No."

"Do us a favor, Joyner, and shut up," Marson said.

"Where's your family?" Joyner asked. Then he looked at Marson. "Get him to tell you where they are."

"Roma," the old man said.

"You understand more English than you're letting on, huh."

The eyes gave no sign of comprehension.

"He knows," Joyner said. "And I bet he can tell us what's on the other side of this fuck'n mountain we're climbing."

"We know what's on the other side," Asch said. "The fucking war."

"I just don't think we should trust him."

"La mia famiglia," the old man said. "Roma."

Joyner kept digging at himself. "Shit. You guys — just remember this son of a bitch was part of the Axis, okay? And he's seventy — which means he was around for Albania and the Africa stuff, at the beginning. Ethiopia — all that."

"What about Ethiopia?" Marson said. "What the hell are you talking about?"

"It goes back ten years and more," Joyner told him. "These guys've been fighting a long time. I'm sure they're sick of it, but

145

some of them are probably sick in other ways."

The old man understood that they were talking about him. He kept smiling, clearly trying to show good will. Marson felt ashamed and tried to soften the old man's anxiety. He nodded at him and then offered him some water from his canteen. The old man took it, keeping one eye on Joyner.

Joyner said, "You don't fool me, pie-zan. I ain't like these guys."

"Molti bambini," Angelo said, smiling and nodding.

"Wouldn't surprise me if you know every word we're saying."

He kept the smile, but glanced away.

The wind suddenly died down once more, and all around them was deep stillness. Beyond the root tangle at the foot of the downed tree, the dead soldier was like another part of the woods. The snow had covered the legs and filled wrinkles in the tunic, and it had gathered at the neck and in the ears. It kept drawing their gaze to it. Nothing stirred anywhere else.

"Shit," Asch said to Joyner. "Think of it as a statue."

"How long do we have to fuck'n stay here," Joyner said, digging at the place on his arm.

"Not much longer," said Marson.

The old man coughed again, and this time it became a fit. He held his hands over his mouth, attempting to muffle the noise. The coughing went on.

"Great. Let's send up a flare," said Joyner. He grabbed a handful of snow and packed it into his sleeve. "Fuck'n freezing. And I've gotta put ice on my fuck'n arm."

Asch stirred suddenly and scrabbled through the snow a few feet away and was sick there, noisily, with a terrible-sounding loud belch. Then he groaned and was sick again. He came back and crouched with his back against the tree trunk. "I didn't even know I was gonna do that."

"You all right now?" Marson asked him.

"I don't know." He indicated the corpse lying only a few feet away. "I can't stop looking at that. I just got a feeling, like a jolt, like a — like a sudden remembering where I am. And I thought of the whore. It got me. Let's get out of here and get a look over the other side and then get our asses back down to the road. Jesus."

"Near," said the old man.

"If he says that one more time I'm gonna blow him to Sardinia," Joyner said.

"Man," Asch said. "Let up a little."

"I don't wanna die on this fucker."

"Stop talking shit," said Corporal Marson. "We're gonna wait another fifteen minutes. Be quiet and listen and maybe we won't die."

Again, they were silent. The quiet stretched on away from them. It was impossible to believe that there was a war on the other side of the hill, beyond whatever hills there were. But then another little breeze stirred, and it brought a sound to them, a distant hum. Marson thought he might be imagining it. Asch said, "What the hell is that?"

Joyner, holding his arm, said, "Planes."

"No," said Marson. "Tanks."

"Jesus Christ. Up here?"

"No."

"Carri armati," the old man said.

"Near?" said Joyner, spitting.

"No, signore."

"Yeah — we'll find out that 'near' means the fuck'n Jerries."

"It *is* tanks," Marson said. "Come on, move out." He indicated for the old man to lead the way.

They followed him, past the body of the dead German, across the corridor of snow and into the trees, up another swale of ground, and then a path down again, more and more steeply, so that several times they

they slid in the snow and had to hold on and pause. There were a large number of foot tracks where they walked now, and they kept low, moving once more from tree to tree with stealth. The old man was doing the same. They had been doing this for some time before it came to Marson to wonder whether he himself had started this or had followed the lead of the old man. He was too exhausted to think. He looked at the moon in the starry sky and understood that they had not yet crossed midnight. At a wide, extended stairlike ledge of rock, he signaled the old man with a tap on his back to stop. They all slid out on the first tier of the ledge to look down. There was another snowfield, perhaps fifty yards across, and the crowding tops of more pines. Beyond that was another mountain, other mountains. The snowfield was heavily marked up with foot tracks, all going away.

"They came through here after the snow stopped," said Marson.

"Near," the old man said, nodding.

Marson turned to Asch and Joyner. "That shot we heard — it was what we left back there. Whatever —"

Asch interrupted him. "It took you until now to figure that out?"

Marson went on, more slowly. "Whatever

they're up to, it's got nothing to do with us. So let's see if we can get a look at what they're running to, from a distance, and then go back down."

"We gotta go *up* again before we go back down," Joyner said.

Marson said, "We'll give them a little time to get farther away."

They moved back off the ledge and down, to the hollow beneath it. A mound of drifted snow hid them and kept them from the stirrings of the frigid air. Marson's clothes were almost dry now, from the outside in, the wind having taken care of the outer surfaces. His underclothes were still soggy and they clung to him in all the wrong ways. The others were suffering the same discomforts. They ate some more rations, and Asch passed his canteen, then filled it with snow and put it back.

"We're gonna have to climb this fucker again, you know," Joyner said.

Asch said, "We know they're going away, don't we?"

"A little farther," said the corporal. "If we get to where we can see down to the road from a distance, we'll know more."

"How much do you wanna know?" Joyner said. He was scratching his arm again, pulling at the snow and using it to freeze the

150

abraded place.

The wind picked up once more, a cold scarf lashing across their faces.

"I want to know enough. What we were sent to know. And shut up."

"Why'd you pick me for this fucker, anyway."

"I didn't pick you. Glick did."

"Glick's a killer," Asch said. "We're soldiers. He's a killer."

"Listen."

They paused. Far away, barely discernible, the wind was carrying another sound. Shooting. It was shooting. Unmistakable. But not a battle or a skirmish. The shots seemed timed — spaced at nearly exact intervals. Each of the men looked at the others, each trying to solve the problem of the sound and what it meant. It occurred to them almost simultaneously that they were hearing executions. Marson nodded at Asch, who was frowning, and then nodding, too. They were certain of it, now. The old man began to mutter, low, a singsong whose words were not even distinguishable as words.

"*Il mio paese,*" he said to Marson. And he put his head down.

"*Paese.*"

"*Amici. Amici del mio cuore.*" The old man

151

put one hand on his chest, over his heart.

"*Amici* — friend," Marson said. "Friend of your heart."

"*Casa mia.* How you say — house."

"Home."

"*Sì.*"

"I'm so sorry."

The old man did not respond. He folded his hands tightly at his thin chest, concentrating very deeply on something in his own thoughts, muttering low again.

"*Assassini,*" the old man said through his bad teeth. "Killers."

They listened and the shooting went on, slow, gaps of a few seconds between shots, a volley each time, a firing squad, and the Germans were apparently shooting a lot of people, lining them up and shooting them down. With each volley the old man uttered a little sound of grief.

"Goddamn," Asch said. "Are they shooting *everybody?*"

"*Vigliacchi. Criminali.*"

"They're shooting criminals?"

"*Sono criminali.*"

"I don't understand what the fuck he's saying," Asch said. "Are they shooting the whole village?"

"*I Tedeschi sono criminali,*" said the old man.

"The Germans are the criminals," Marson said.

"Vigliacchi! Sì. Cowards. *Tedeschi."* He spit.

They listened. There were two more volleys, and then a pause, then two more. It went on.

"Goddamn," Asch said. "Goddamn."

There was a long pause. And then it began again.

Marson said, "What the hell."

*"God*damn them," Asch said suddenly, loud. "Oh, goddamn them." He stood and looked out over the mound of drifted snow at the marked wide field and the tops of trees and shouted, "You goddamn motherfucking sons of bitches! I'll kill every fucking one of you!"

"But who are they shooting?" Joyner said. "Are they killing the whole fucking village? What the fuck."

"Ebrei," said the old man.

"Ebrei," Asch said. "I heard that at Palermo. *Ebrei.* Hebrews. He's talking about Jews." He looked out at the marked-up snowfield, the black tops of the trees. "They're shooting Jews?"

They had heard rumors of what the Germans were doing in the north. They had not believed the rumors.

Joyner was digging at his arm, his mouth

153

pulled back in a grimace.

"Ebrei," said the old man, looking down. *"Sì."*

Asch had even talked about atrocity propaganda from the first war, having heard similar stories from his grandfather.

"Why would they — ?" Marson said. And his nausea came back, silencing him. He turned and sat down in the snow, leaning against the rock wall. Beside him, Asch's voice had spilled over into a kind of manic muttering.

"That's — that's bullshit. That's bullshit. They're shooting partisans. Something —"

"What the fuck," Joyner said. "What the *fuck.*"

"Ebrei," the old man said. *"Amici."* His eyes kept brimming. *"Amici."*

They heard another volley. It made them all wince. Marson tried to pray, murmuring the Lord's Prayer. He kept repeating the phrase in his mind, *deliver us from evil, deliver us from evil . . .*

"That's bullshit," Asch said, again, and then again. And then he murmured something in another language: *"Yisgadal v'yiskadash sh'mei rabbaw."* He took a quick, sobbing breath. *"B'allmaw dee v'raw chir'usei v'yamlich malchusei, b'chayeichon, uv'yomeichon, uv'chayei d'chol beis yis-*

roel . . ."

"What're you saying?" Joyner asked.

Asch looked at him as if he had been startled out of sleep. "Nothing," he said. "I don't believe it." He gestured with a tilting of his head toward the direction of the shots, the village. "But they do."

Joyner did not take his eyes away.

"It's called Kaddish, okay? Mourner's Prayer. Prayer for the dead."

Joyner sat back and began concentrating on his arm again. "Goddamn," he said. "Oh god*damn.*"

"I learned it as a kid," Asch told them. Then he muttered again: *"Y'hei shlawmaw rabbaw min sh'mayaw, v'chayim awleinu v'al kol yisroel."*

"What's it mean?" Marson asked him.

"Yeah," Joyner said, almost like a challenge, except that he had a forlorn look in his eyes. "Tell us what it's saying."

Asch sighed, and the tears ran down his cheeks. "Ah — God. Look. It means — I don't know what it means. It means you say it for the dead." He gasped, choked, held his fist to his mouth, then took it away — his hand dropped to his side. "It means whatever it means when you can't —" He sniffled and ran his wrist across his face. "Ah. Man," he said. "Words. Goddamn."

155

They were all silent then. Asch murmured the prayer under his breath.

Each volley made them recoil. And it went on, and on. Perhaps an hour of it while they looked out at the snowfield with its tracks leading away. The sky above them was beautiful, dark and full of stars, with small white tufts and high thin ribbons of cirrus, gleaming at the edges with the moon. The whole sky was colored with that light, and the stars sparkled in it like gemstones strewn across a vast bed.

"What're you gonna report now about the Kraut whore?" Joyner said suddenly, low.

Asch didn't answer him for a moment. Then: "I'm gonna report a murder."

"No shit. After this?"

"Yes," Asch said. "*Especially* after this. *Especially* after this, goddamn it."

"She was a fucking Nazi, Saul. Christ. How clear do you need it to be?"

Another volley quieted them. Asch sat very still, staring out. Then he was sick, putting his head down between his knees.

Marson watched him and kept trying to pray. He could not find the words. Each time there was a volley, the sound of it and what it meant rose up in him, facing at him, a wall against which his own soul could only collide in unbelief. He searched for something to feel other than the sickness and the vacancy of not being able to process the fact of what the sounds meant. It was all a blankness like the blankness of a field of snow where no human tracks have ever been made. And the world before his eyes *was* beautiful, like a painting, and the stars sparkled in the sky.

"Maybe they're shooting officers, like the guy back up the hill," Joyner said, and then seemed to choke.

Asch indicated the old man. "You heard him."

"Murderers," the old man said, distinctly, like someone well versed in the language. He looked at Marson and said it again, clearly. "Murderers."

"God," Marson said. "Ah, God."

In another moment, the volleys stopped. And the silence became freighted with waiting for the next one, which didn't come.

"I can't stand this anymore," Joyner said suddenly. He stood and hurled his carbine down into the snowfield — it made no sound, dropping in and leaving the imprint of itself — then ripped his field jacket off, and his blouse, so that his arms were bare. He knelt and stuck his bad arm down in the snow, all the way to the shoulder.

"Joyner, for Christ's sweet sake," Asch

157

said, wiping the back of his hand across his face, sniffling.

Joyner didn't move, but kept the arm down in the snow, the whole arm.

"Come on, Joyner," said the corporal. "Don't make me have to report you."

"Hey, don't report me. Shoot me."

"Stop this. Get your gear and your stuff together. We're moving out."

They waited. He wept a little, moving the bad arm in the snowdrift, as if he had lost something and was feeling around for it. Finally he stood again and wiped the snow from himself, crying, cursing. Asch handed him his shirt. Asch buttoned it for him because in the few moments the snow had rendered Joyner's hand too numb to function. He let it dangle at his side while Asch worked on him.

"I gotta get off this fucker," Joyner said. "Jesus Christ. We gotta get away from all this shit. It's shit. I gotta get back off this motherfucker of a mountain and out of this fucking terrible place."

Marson said, "Go get your weapon."

"I don't care what you tell them down on the road. I don't care if they court-martial me. Fuck it. I mean it."

"Let's just get this over with, Joyner. Okay?"

158

Joyner walked out onto the snowfield and made his way across to the weapon. And he brought it back, head down. He stood with the others, carbine in one hand, scratching that forearm with the other hand.

"Let's go," Marson said.

"I'm staying here," said Joyner, still looking down. "I'll be here when you come back through. And I don't care what you do and I don't care what you say."

Marson waited.

"Near," the old man said, low. It was clear that he had understood what was happening.

"Joyner, don't do this," Marson said.

"I'll cover your back, Corporal. I'm not going over there."

Marson felt an urge, nearly irresistible, to strike him. But they were in this space together now, having been through the sounds from the village, having been faced with this something so far beyond their own worst expectations of themselves or of the world, even a world at war. It was a strange, sorrowful moment, suffused almost with a tenderness. He had to work to put it down in himself. He took a breath, and then turned to Asch. "You're a witness to this," he said. He was calling it up from all his training. "And I believe the penalty for desertion is death."

Asch looked at him with unconcealed surprise.

"Got it?" Marson said.

"It's not desertion if I'm covering your back," said Joyner, a pleading note in his voice.

"It's desertion if you disobey an order to march in a combat situation."

"*È molto vicino*. Good — near."

"Tell him to shut up," Joyner said. "Goddamn it, I mean it. I don't like his language. Tell him to just shut the fuck up."

"I'm telling *you* to shut up," Marson said. And he turned to Asch again. "You're a witness."

"I'm that," said Asch. "I *am* that — Christ."

"We're going on," Marson said to Joyner. "You can stay here and suffer the consequences or you can fall in. If you fall in, we never mention it." He gestured for Angelo to lead on, and started with him around the snow mound, descending again. After a few paces, he stopped. Asch and Joyner were coming behind them.

"*Molto vicino,*" the old man said.

They kept going. Not talking, following him. There were no openings in the trees, and the ground kept dipping. They kept descending. You couldn't see out for the tree branches, all pines now, thick and drooping with snow. The air was colder on this side of the mountain, or seemed so. At last they came to a shoulder, at the end of which they could see a narrow plain, opening out below, with the river running far off to the left, and the road and several farm fields ending in the cluster of buildings and houses that was, no doubt, Angelo's unfortunate village. Beyond that were foothills and the other mountains. On the road, going away, several tanks rolled along, panzers, and, looking through the scope, you could see the troops marching alongside them. It looked like an orderly retreat.

Nineteen

They had turned around and were climbing again, going back up to the crest, past the marks of their descending. They got to the snowfield in front of the long terracelike ledge, and when Saul Asch paused to adjust a damp fold in the front of his field jacket, something hit him in the back.

As he toppled forward, they all heard the shot.

It came from very far off. Asch went over like a felled tree. The others scurried for the drift of snow under the ledge. They made it there and got down and stayed down, and waited. Marson looked out over the snow hillock. Asch lay still and quiet, on his stomach in the open, face to one side.

"Jesus, Jesus, Jesus, Jesus," Joyner kept saying under his breath. The old man moaned and lay on his side, his cloak pulled high over his head.

"Where'd it come from?" Marson said.

"I don't know," Joyner said. "Christ. Behind us. Way off."

"A sniper?"

"Oh, Jesus, Jesus, Jesus. I knew it. They're following us."

"No, it's a sniper."

"Are you sure?" Joyner sighted with his carbine, sweeping the panorama of the moonlit space.

Out in the field, Asch moved, seemed about to try and get up. Marson called to him. "Stay absolutely still, Saul. Don't move. If he knows you're alive he'll shoot again. Hold still!"

Joyner said, "We can't leave him there."

"Shut up, we're not going to."

"He'll die if we don't get to him."

The moon shone, terribly bright in a mostly clear and starry sky, and Asch's shape in the field was not moving. Everything beyond him looked as still as a photograph.

Joyner became worried that the enemy could be working around the snowfield in the trees. He kept thinking he heard footfalls, and twice he whirled, ready to shoot.

"I'm telling you it's a sniper," Marson said.

The old man repeated the word in English. Then moaned and crossed himself.

Marson looked out at Asch where he lay, a shadow outlined with silver light. There was so much light. It hurt the eyes to look at it. But there were little moving silvery clouds in the sky. A small tuft was drifting slow on a trajectory to block the moon. It might cover it, or part of it, for a little space. "I'm coming to get you, Asch. Just stay still."

They waited. The little cloud missed the moon. The old man whimpered and seemed again to be saying something, some chant in Italian, repeating it over and over. The cold felt solid now, the wind battering them. "I'm gonna go get him," Marson said.

"Jesus, do you think he's dead?"

"I'm not leaving him there."

"I didn't say that," Joyner got out. And then he seemed to think more deeply into what had been said. "Hey, fuck you, Marson."

"Just stay put," Marson told him. "When I start, cover me."

"Cover you how? The fucker's probably on another mountain."

They peered at the snowfield and the trees beyond, trying to decide where the shot must have come from. Because there had been no more shooting, they knew this was indeed a sniper, a straggler left behind to delay pursuit. And probably he was still out there somewhere.

The wind lifted more snow, and as a cloud shadow passed across the field, Marson got to his feet, his legs trembling as with some nerve weakness, and made for where Asch lay. He took one shaky step, and then another, and another. He felt as though he might collapse any second. The moon, even in the little fold of cloud, was still dazzling, the field too bright, and there were all the foot tracks of human progress across it, and he thought of it that way — oddly, like a reflection in someone else's mind, even while he ran, even while he felt the terror and the certainty of eyes on him — that here were the signs of human habitation in the open snowy expanse, as if it were the surface of some ice planet. It seemed to him that the stars beyond the clouds and the moon were making their own light. He pushed through the crusting snow, wishing for perfect darkness, feeling himself exposed, watched, followed in sights, a figure in crosshairs, moving in a zigzag, expecting any moment to feel the piercing of the bullet, and to feel it before the sound reached him. But he got to Asch and pitched forward in the snow, his face only inches from Asch's face.

Asch lay quite still, eyes closed, the snow

adhering to his cheeks. His mouth was slightly open, and snow had got into it. Crystals of it glistened in his hair. Marson thought of the dead German. He reached over and got Asch's helmet, which had flown from him when he fell.

"Saul," he said, into the snow-spattered face.

Asch opened his eyes. "I'm shot," he said. "Christ." He started to cry. "Oh, Jesus Christ. I'm shot."

"Listen to me," Marson said. "Can you get up?"

The other man gave him a look of profound exasperation. "Yeah. You wanna dance? We'll waltz out of here. They'll never know what happened."

"If I put your arm over my neck, can you help walk?"

"Just get me out of here, man. I'm shot. Goddamn. I'm shot. Oh, Jesus Christ." He was crying again.

Marson got to his knees, shouldered Asch's carbine alongside his own, and then lifted him, standing, using his hip and managing to get the other's arm across his own neck while still holding the helmet. He staggered with the weight, calling on what felt like the last of his strength, trying to run, aware that snipers watched for the ones trying to help. He felt the immense certainty that he would be shot in the next instant. It made his bowels drop. His voice went out from him, a cry, like a cry of pain. But nothing struck. He was struggling with the other man in the moonlit field and nothing came from the shooter in the distance.

"I can't feel my fucking legs, man." Asch sobbed. "I'll never see my child, you know? Christ. I'm gonna die now, right? Isn't that right, Marson? I'm gonna die. Oh, Christ, I can't feel my legs."

Marson carried him, stumbling in the heavy snow, toward the protection of the ledge, beyond the hillock of driven snow with their frantic tracks all over it. The knowledge that he would not hear the shot until it hit him made him groan and push through, panic rising in him, the sound of the snow breaking at his feet too loud, everything pounding, everything shouting with the not-sound of the bullet he felt coming at him, and he was down at last, out of the clearing at last, below the level of the hill, under the ledge, gasping, and Joyner crouched there with the old man, both of them staring out at the place from which he and Asch had come. There were no other shots.

TWENTY

Joyner put a blanket down in a flat dry place under the ledge. Asch lay partly on his right side. He moaned, half conscious now. The other two worked on him, removing his pack and pulling at his field jacket and blouse to get a look at the wound. The bullet had entered his rib cage, missing bone, about eight to ten inches above his hip on the left side, and exited a little down from that and perhaps an inch toward the middle of his lower abdomen. It had traveled a long way and did not seem to have broken bone. The exit wound was slightly larger than the entrance wound, and the blood kept coming there, a spreading black stain in the moonlight. Joyner and Marson kept trying to stanch it with gauzes from Marson's first-aid kit, and then from Joyner's. They pressed their hands to it, and Marson worried about what might be approaching from the other side of the field. But the old man was watching, and also watching the struggle to stop Asch's bleeding.

"I'm freezing," Asch said. "I'm so fucking cold."

Marson tried to cover him, but you couldn't work to stop the bleeding if you couldn't see the wounds, and now the entrance wound began bleeding, too, filling with blood and then flowing over. The blanket was soaked. They kept working the wounds.

"It's not stopping," Asch sobbed. "Christ. I'm emptying out."

"It is stopping," Joyner told him. "It is."

They worked on, feeling the inimical presence in the moon-haunted dark all around them.

"I didn't do anything," Asch said, low, beginning to cry. "I was a nice guy. I never hurt anybody intentionally, I swear it."

"Shut up," said Joyner. "It's stopping. We'll wrap you up and take you down and you'll be out of the fuck'n war."

"I'm scared, Benny. It's bad, isn't it. I can't stop shivering."

Joyner was silent, working hard to make the bleeding stop. Marson stood and looked out at the field and the sky. Asch's breathing was becoming faster. The entrance wound had stopped bleeding. Another blast of the wind made him realize that the man's bare flesh was exposed. He knelt and tried to cover his back with the bloody field jacket. Joyner was still working the exit wound, murmuring, "It's slowing down. Slowing down now. It's gonna be fine. It's stopping."

"It's starting to hurt," Asch said. "Oh, Christ help me. It hurts bad."

"It's stopped bleeding," Joyner said. "The cold's good. It's really slowing it down."

"I'm freezing. God."

"It's doing good. Almost completely stopped now. I swear."

"I need something for the pain, though. Give me something for the pain."

There were morphine syringes in the first-aid kit. Marson pulled the seal from one and stuck it into Asch's thigh.

"Give him another one," Joyner said.

Marson did so.

"I didn't mean anything," Asch moaned.

The corporal saw Angelo watching all of this, and watching the field, too. The old man's face looked changed, the odd marks in the forehead showing in the shadowy light, the black eyes simply taking everything in. Marson had an unpleasant foreboding sense of having missed something about him.

Asch wept softly, apologizing for the noise. "I didn't mean anything. I'm sorry, fellas."

"You're out of the war," Joyner said. "You lucky son of a bitch."

"But God, Benny. There's so much blood."

"We've all got gallons of it," Joyner told him. "Plenty to spare. I bled as much from a head cut in a football game."

"I got it all over," said Asch as if worried about the mess.

"It's stopping," Joyner told him. "You take a vial of blood you'd donate and spill it and it'll look about like this."

"I spilled a lot of blood, fellas." Asch sobbed.

For a little space, then, they were all quiet. There was only the sound of the wounded soldier's breathing and moaning. "If I could quit shivering. God — I knew we'd get it. I knew it. I knew we'd get it on this fucking piece-of-shit mountain. We were cursed from the start."

Through it all, the old man seemed simply to regard the others in their trouble while continuing to keep watch on the snowfield. It seemed to Marson that he had the demeanor of someone who had no fear for himself anymore. He seemed almost detached. It was disturbing, and Marson marked it, deciding that it would be wise to watch him more closely. It was possible that instead of keeping watch for an approaching enemy, he was looking for a possible rescuer. The thought blew through the corporal like a blast of icy wind, and he stepped over to the old man and looked out at the field. "Do you see something?" he asked. *"Capeesh?"*

The old man shook his head. Something about him appeared faintly arrogant now, as if he could not be bothered to fear or respect these armed boys he was with in their trouble. Marson thought of this and it was as if he were briefly inside the other's mind. He stood close, trying to see into the darkness of the eyes. The moon did not lend enough light to see the irises. But Marson was reasonably certain that he was not imagining the feeling. He said, *"Tedesco?"*

"*Italiano,* signore."

"Guide, right?"

"Guida, sì."

"*Tedeschi* out there?" Marson pointed.

"Tedeschi — no. *Nessun tedesco. Nessuno che veda. Niente."*

"You take us back down this mountain." Corporal Marson wanted it to have the force of a command.

But the old man looked at him blankly

172

and seemed to be waiting for him to falter somehow. *Non capisco.*

"Fellas?" Asch said suddenly. "Fellas?"

"We're here," Joyner told him.

"Fellas, I can't move my legs."

"I'm sure it missed your spine," Joyner said.

"I can't move my legs, fellas."

Joyner grabbed his ankle. "Can you feel that?"

"Feel what?"

He looked at Marson.

"Oh, Christ — Christ. I can't feel my legs."

"It'll pass," Joyner told him. He was still working the exit wound. Marson watched the old man, and the trees. He used the scope to pan the expanse of disturbed snow and the far tree line. He saw no movement anywhere.

"You're gonna be thanking God for this wound," Joyner said to Asch.

He got the bleeding stopped at last. But there was still the problem of the legs. It was strange that the legs were as they were, since the bullet had missed the spine altogether, by several inches. It had exited on a line inches to the left side. Nothing of it would have broken off or splintered. There was no danger of injuring the spine with

173

motion, or there wasn't any that Marson could think of, and Joyner, who Stateside had done a few weeks of training as a medic, said there certainly wasn't. Joyner attributed the loss of feeling to shock and said he was practically certain feeling would return as soon as Asch's blood pressure rose to normal. He said as much to Asch, speaking with certainty, and Asch thanked him, and then lapsed into semiconsciousness. "Billy?" he said, loud, so that his voice carried. "Where's the toothpaste. Somebody took the toothpaste."

Joyner said, "I've got it, Saul."

Asch seemed greatly relieved. "Ah, thanks, Billy. You're a good brother." He wept a little more. "I should've given you that baseball glove. You should've seen what I saw, Billy. In the Sahara Desert. Can't get it out of my mind." Joyner was working to get the bandages tight around the wound.

They could not be certain there was no internal bleeding. From this angle, it looked like the bullet could have perforated part of the bowel. Joyner leaned into Marson and told him this. Marson saw the old man watching them.

"Father?" Asch said, low, and was gone again.

They wrapped him in bandages from all

three kits. The old man watched them and kept glancing at the row of trees bordering the field on the right side.

"You waiting for something there?" Marson asked him again.

The old man did not know he was being addressed.

"Angelo."

He turned, startled.

"Anything you're expecting to see out there?"

"Non capisco," Angelo said.

They closed Asch's field jacket, and after a wait of a few tense minutes, scanning the prospect of the field in the bath of moonlight and the trees lining it, they began again their trek across the brow of the mountain and toward the way down. Marson carried Asch over his back, holding one arm at the wrist and, with his left hand through the legs, gripping the thick thigh. Joyner carried the carbines and two packs. The old man led them, carrying the other pack. They moved through the trees. Several times they had to stop and listen, and rest. They made very slow progress. And all the time the air got colder, the wind more piercing. They kept moving, and Marson's legs burned, his sides caught, he couldn't breathe out fully. The blister on his heel sent white-hot pain all the way to his hip. He would stagger the few feet to the next tree, the next shape or outcropping of rock that might provide cover from a distant shooter, and he continued trying to pray, the God he believed in beginning to feel like the immensity itself all around him. And through it all, he kept sensing someone trying to hold him in crosshairs.

When they arrived at the site of the camp with the dead German in it, they got to the other side of the downed tree and tried to rest awhile. Marson set Asch down carefully in the snow, so that he lay partly on his side again. Joyner looked to see if the wounds were bleeding more. They were not. The two soldiers ranged themselves on either side of Asch and breathed the cold air, and waited for the strength to continue. Asch was unconscious, dreaming something. He mentioned Billy several times, and Africa, in a jumble of words. Marson did not want to think that in his delirium he might be reliving the burning tank.

The wind picked up again, but the snow had mostly frozen, a crust of solidness that their boots had to break through with each step they took. It had drifted over the body of the German officer almost entirely — the body made only a human-shaped mound, now, with a little sharp corner of frozen cloth, a shirt collar, jutting out of it where the neck would be.

Marson drank from his canteen and realized the old man was watching him. He offered the canteen, and the old man drank deeply. If the sniper was pursuing them, he could pick them off one by one. The thought brought Marson to a crouch, peering out past the body-shaped mound, for any sign of movement. The old man handed him the canteen and got down behind the tree, knees up, arms wrapped around them.

"I don't think we'll ever know who it was or what it was," Joyner said.

"They send stragglers," Marson said. "He probably shot once and went on with the retreat."

"Or he's fuck'n hunting us."

Marson looked out. The trees and shadows appeared motionless as printed images. The wind had paused.

"It's not so bad, the cold, as long as the wind isn't blowing." Joyner offered his canteen to Asch, who had stirred but had not quite awakened. He took it back and drank of it, little sips, and then he made a gagging noise. "Sorry," he said.

"You all right?" Marson asked him.

"I'm sick. It was a lot of blood. I don't do

blood too well, you know? I couldn't make it through medic training because of it."

The field, which looked like a lane between the two rows of trees, was unchanged. "What time do you think it is?"

"Not much past midnight."

The old man coughed and sputtered and rubbed his mouth. He laid his head back against the tree and closed his eyes.

"I've got an idea," Joyner said.

Marson turned to him.

"Let's set the Kraut up to look like one of us, with a carbine. Lean him against the tree or something. If there's a sniper on our tail, maybe he'll take a shot at our dead friend. You know? It can be a warning for us."

Marson said, "What if he shoots us while we're setting it up?"

"We're in some tree shade here. Be a tough shot."

"You want to take that chance?"

"If there's something I can do to get rid of the feeling somebody's drawing a fuck'n bead on me all the way down this fucker."

"Okay, then let's do it."

They stood at the same time, and the old man stood, too. Marson noticed that he had put Asch's pack on, and the straps hung from it. Probably it provided some warmth for him. When Marson tried to catch his eye, to communicate, the old man simply looked away.

"No move," Corporal Marson said. "Stay."

The old man waited. Marson stepped over to him and gestured for him to get down. Asch moaned and then turned slightly and raised his head. "Robert?"

"We're gonna set up a decoy," Marson said to him.

"We're not down the mountain?"

"Not yet."

"I knew it. I'm bleeding again, too. I can feel it."

Marson knelt down, pulled back the field jacket, and looked at the bandaged place. He saw no stain of blood on it. "You're not bleeding now," he said.

"I can feel it," said Asch. "Inside."

"Stay still," Marson said, and again he gestured to the old man to get down. Joyner had already moved to the other side of the tree, had already stepped into the water of the little stream, which the snow had covered. It had not quite frozen over. He cursed and sat down. "Fuck'n ice. God-damn it. I'll get frostbite now and lose a fuck'n foot."

Marson walked over and helped him stand. They stood on the other side of the tree, in the moonlight, and they realized it at the same time, looking out along the snow lane, fearing the shot they would not hear.

TWENTY-ONE

It took a long time, working to free the corpse, breaking the frozen crust with their entrenching tools, and then scooping at the snow with their hands to get to the outline of it. Ice had formed over the face, and the hands had frozen so solidly that the fingers would not come free. Joyner chopped through four of the fingers with the sharp end of the tool to free the left hand. He gagged and coughed, moving off a few feet, to the trees. He kept gasping. "This is awful," he said. "Goddamn."

"Come on," said Marson.

"I'm sick."

The old man coughed and moved out from the tree, holding Asch's pack. *"Che cosa state facendo?* What that you do?"

"Down," Marson said to him, gesturing.

Joyner made his way back to the body and began tearing at the snow around the legs. He kept muttering, cursing, glancing at the open space in its bath of lunar brightness. Marson got down to help him, and the old man simply crouched and watched them.

Somehow they got the other hand free without damaging it. Twice they stopped, and listened, and Joyner went and checked on Asch, who was by turns fitfully awake and unconscious. The old man went back to the tree trunk and sat against it, with Asch's pack behind him for a cushion. He rocked back and forth in the cold, arms clasping his upraised knees, staring at Asch, and intermittently he would raise himself and fix his gaze on the open area of ground.

The body was rock solid, stiff, and much heavier than either of the two soldiers imagined it could be. Finally the old man had to come around the tree and help. They got it upright, but the arms were out-stretched, as though it were reaching for the clear, star- and moon-bright sky. The shadow it made across the trampled surface of snow looked like the shadow of a statue. "I never thought I'd ever wish for rain," Joyner said. "Something other than this fuck'n moon. Jesus."

They lifted the body like a big solid log, carried it to one of the trees just beyond the campsite, and propped it there. Marson broke through the crust of snow and piled some of it around the feet for support. There were about eleven inches between the feet, the legs having spread slightly in the toppling over from being shot.

"Nobody's gonna be fooled by this," Joyner wheezed. He stood there trying to gain his breath back.

"Can we get the arms down?"

"Solid as stone."

"Wrap your blanket roll around him."

"Have to use Asch's. Mine's covered with blood."

Asch's was also covered with blood, and stiffening in the cold. They got it to conform to the shape of the body. Then they stepped back a little to look at it in the dimness. It looked as though the soldier were trying to climb the tree.

"Let's wrap the blanket around the arms and the tree," Marson said, "and leave the head out."

They tried this. Joyner was gasping for air and coughing, gagging. Marson kept track of the old man out of the corner of his eye. When they got the body tied, they stepped back again to survey their work. Now it looked as though the figure were hugging the tree.

"Shit," Joyner said. "It's gonna have to do."

Marson put Asch's helmet on it. He had to pack the helmet with snow. Joyner emptied the clip from Asch's carbine and lay it in the fold of the blanket near the chest line. Through it all they had to keep pausing to listen.

"Well," Marson said, gazing at it. "I don't know."

"It looks like a stiff tied to a fuck'n tree."

"A mannequin," Marson said. "But maybe from a distance."

Asch made a noise of choking, and they hurried around to him. Saliva had gathered in the back of his throat. He coughed it up, looked at them, muttered something about the cold, and began to murmur, crying. They couldn't make any of it out. Then he lapsed back into unconsciousness.

Marson stationed himself near the base of the tree and scoped the lane between the rows of trees. Joyner sat beside him with his back to the trunk. The old man faced Joyner, crouched low, gazing at Asch, who kept twitching and moaning, but did not come to. Marson felt the searing pain in his foot. He waited for the strength to move. There were more clouds now, a wide shoreline-looking expanse of them, advancing incrementally from the east. Soon it would be as dark as it had been in the rain.

Marson indicated this to Joyner, who nodded.

They got Asch across Joyner's back, and with the old man carrying Asch's pack, they started again, making their way slowly, torturously down, and Marson did not remember it being this steep at this part of the climb. But the snow held them some, the crust of it breaking with each stride they made and then hugging their thighs. The old man took them back down the path on which he'd first led them, and at one bend in it, he paused, and looked to his left, expectation on his face. He peered through the trees.

"You see something?" Marson asked him.

"Niente." But there had been that look.

When they came to the place where they had seen the buck, they moved to the lee of a big tree and paused again. Asch remained unconscious but breathing. The old man put the pack down and leaned on it, sighing.

Marson looked at him, certain that there had been a subtle change in him; now he seemed like someone full of anticipation. His manner was that of a man waiting in ambush.

"Angelo," Marson told him, smiling. "If you do anything to guide them to us I'll shoot you before I take the first shot at them. *Capeesh?*"

"*Guida,*" the old man said, nodding. He smiled but then seemed to think better of it. He had his arms wrapped about himself, leaning against Asch's pack.

"I said from the start I don't trust him." Joyner was winded. His words came with a rasping. "Christ. He'd do it, too. You see it now, too. Right? You think he's Fascist, too."

"I don't know what I think," Marson said.

"*Non sono fascista,*" said Angelo.

They waited. Joyner drank from his canteen and then, after a hesitation that demonstrated his distrust, offered it to the old man, who had just put a handful of snow in his mouth. The old man shook his head. "*Grazie,* no."

In the next half minute of silence they heard a shot, echoing across the silent snow and the blackness of the trees, from very far.

Twenty-Two

Sound carries farther at this height, Marson told himself. The shot was behind them. He believed it had come from there. "I'm going to double back," he told Joyner. "And take him out."

"Naw, look," Joyner said. "Let's just get back down off this fucker."

"We can't move fast enough. He'll pick us off. He'll get where he can see us all and he'll pick us off."

"I don't think so. I think we should get down to the road fast."

Marson thought a moment. "Let Angelo take you down. Just keep going. I'll catch up to you either way."

The old man stared from one to the other of them. But then he pointed back up the mountain. *"Tedeschi,"* he said.

"Yeah. Get going," Marson said.

Asch moaned.

"This cold will save his life," Joyner said.

"He can't bleed like he would in warmer conditions, I know that."

"Get him down this mountain. I mean it. I'll follow. I can follow the snow trail."

Joyner shook his head. "I got a bad feeling."

"We've gotta know anyway what's trailing us. If it's a regiment, they'll need to know down on the road, right?"

"It's a sniper. I think he probably won't come much farther."

"Just do this for me," Marson said. "Take Asch and go." He looked at the old man. "Down the mountain. *Capeesh?*"

"*Sì,*" the old man said. But clearly he did not understand anything, and only meant to show his loyalty.

Marson indicated Asch, and Joyner, and then he pointed down the mountain. *"Guida."*

"Oh," the old man said, almost eagerly. "*Sì.* Yes. Yes."

"Sorry," Asch mumbled, not quite conscious.

"Okay, we're going down," Joyner said to the old man. "You take one false move and you're dead. *Morto. Capeesh?*"

Angelo looked frightened.

Marson indicated the direction, and gestured again. "Down."

"*Si*. Yes."

He moved off. The old man watched him go. Joyner was doing something with Asch, and Marson saw that he had removed Asch's watch. He went on, wending slowly back through the trees, keeping to the right of the path and going from tree to tree, skirting the ground they had already covered but remaining within clear sight of it, moving very slowly, stopping frequently to listen to the woods. Around him the moonlight began to fail, the shoreline-bright mass of cloud having come over, thin at first, so that the moon shone behind it, but thickening, darkening. The woods seemed more dense in the gloom. At one point it came over him like revelation that he was in Italy, alone, in woods, in the middle of the longest night of his life, and there was someone out there with a scope rifle, hunting him. He stood against a big tree, breathing the odor of its heavy bark, and thought of the pain in his heel. It hurt worse all the time, and yet he could not quite get his mind around it as pain. This that he felt now, stalking the dark, expecting every second to be shot, this was the kind of strain that overmastered the physical discomforts he was suffering, and there was still the cold, the freeze at his fingertips and at the ends of his toes, the shivering, and the feeling of wanting simply to lie down and rest, even knowing that to rest was to die. He could not conjure the slightest image of his own life before this moment, this black quiet, with the terror of any motion or sound, and the sting in his lungs, the shakiness of the muscles in his lower back and his legs.

All for thee, most sacred heart of Jesus.

The words had no meaning. There existed nothing anymore but these woods, this deep stillness. His senses were sharper than they had ever been, and yet he could not think of anything but the darkness and what could be hiding in it. He moved in the blackness like a cat, searching for a place to wait in ambush.

He came to within a few yards of the campsite and saw the corpse lying next to the tree. This fact thrilled him. He got down on his knees, behind a stone outcropping, and waited. After a few minutes of listening, and panning the lane with the scope, he got to where he could see the corpse, but he could not tell in the dark if there had been a hit. He was a few feet away from the downed tree's root system, and he got below the line of it, moving closer to the slight depression in the snow where the fire had been. It had grown too dark to be sure of anything. He simply waited now, reasonably certain that a bullet had knocked the corpse over — the ruse had worked perfectly — and the corpse must have dropped like a shot man. The sniper, if he were indeed following, would then come forward, keeping his distance, moving with the deliberateness of his kind. It felt that way to Marson, as if he were seeking to stop some species, a creature occurring in nature.

The dark was nearly complete. The possibility existed that the sniper had moved beyond this little square of ground, and so it was necessary to try watching in all directions. Marson turned slowly, looking through the almost useless scope. The sense that the sniper may have got by him fed his terror. And it was terror: a deep, black, nerve-tic distress so pervasive that it was hardly aware of itself. Marson stared out at the night in a freezing, fixed gaze of expectation. The darkness yielded no sound. The wind had died. The air grew colder all the time. The line of trees, left and right, the open lane, all of it seemed to be fading out of existence as light left the sky.

Once or twice, over the next minutes, he believed that the corpse moved, or sighed, or took in air. His mind began playing tricks on him. He saw another deer and almost shot at it. The sound of the hooves piercing the snow crust startled him so badly that he let go a little cry from the bottom of his throat. The deer went on. The woods grew silent again. The cold changed in increments of freezing, everything turning to ice. The condensation of his breath froze on his lips. He was beginning to believe that the night would yield up nothing and this had all been a waste. Certainly Joyner and the old man must be well down the mountain, with their cargo. He saw in his mind the look on Asch's face as the bleeding went on, and he knew he should feel sorry for him. He *had* felt sorry for him, and for everyone in the world. But he did not feel it now. He could not find any sense of Asch as another someone. It was as if he were an idea, only a word on someone's lips, a concept. In his mind's eye, he saw the little cracked photograph of his own daughter, and it meant nothing to him. It was a photograph, insubstantial as thought. The waiting was changing him, emptying him, draining all the human elements, as if his spirit were bleeding. He tried to picture Helen, his father and mother, the street, the *surround,* as he had seen it on that last day. He could not call it up. He could not begin to imagine it. The memory of it all was breaking up, dissolving, being effaced awfully. He could see quite clearly the eyes filled with wonder of the dying soldier, the woman's smudged calves. He had become a pair of eyes, staring, two hands on a rifle. A cold watchfulness, shivering in the wind, waiting.

He had not really thought through how he would proceed when he encountered the sniper, what sort of action he might take. He did not know if he was capable of a shot from ambush, and this would have to be just that. He tried imagining himself through it, as he had often imagined himself through pitching to one hitter or another, when he was a good baseball player and there were stupid, trivial things to worry about. He could not see himself through it. He tried to call up the longing he had felt to have his life back again, and he had felt it for so long, and that was gone, too, now. He told himself that he would never complain about anything in his life, if he could take his life out of here, home from this cold dark country with its hills and valleys and mountains, its bad weather. But these were just words, just noises in the mind.

And sleep began to come over him, with stealth, like a kind of nerve-killing predator, closing him down. He nodded off once, caught himself, straightened a little and tightened his grip on the carbine, then nodded off again. His head came against the rough bark of a thick root, and he jolted awake, amazed at the power of this drowsiness, even knowing that he could pay for it with his life. His eyelids were so heavy, so heavy. He took a handful of the snow and put it on his face, felt the intense sting of it, trying to recover his senses. And very quickly the drowse began again. He knelt and pulled at tendrils of the tree's root system, for exercise. Again, he put snow on his face. He saw himself standing in the clearing, and the deer were all around him, and he was falling far.

He woke almost shouting, holding the whimper back. The field had not changed. The night had not changed. He did not know how long he had been asleep, or if indeed he *had* been asleep, until he remembered the deer surrounding him, and the wide clearing he had stood in.

He had no sense of time, and now he had no sense of how long he had been watching the slow progress of a darker shape in the darkness, about a hundred yards from the little campsite, coming along just at the line of the trees, with the open snowfield to the right. He looked at the figure through the scope, but the glass was fogged now. He attempted to spit on the lens but could not produce enough saliva, so he put it in the snow and wiped it off, then raised it and found that he had lost the shape. He tried to see it again in the darkness and could not find it. He was ready to believe that he had been mistaken about what he saw, that it had been nothing more than another deer. He scanned the field again, the line of trees, and saw no moving thing. He put the scope down, and stared. Nothing. He waited, and felt the sleepiness again, and then saw motion, unmistakable, like the darkness itself moving. But it was a shape *in* the darkness, and he was immediately wide awake. It was no deer.

TWENTY-THREE

The man seemed faintly unconcerned with what might be waiting for him, though he was paying some attention to the darker places in the trees. His attitude was that of someone being cautious without fully believing that caution was necessary.

Marson carefully, as soundlessly as he could, attached the scope to his carbine, then got to his knees behind the downed tree, and drew a bead on him.

Not quite gradually, but with a sensation of a slow widening of himself, he felt a lessening of tension, as if something had been released in his blood, a drug, preventing him from feeling what he had felt only seconds before. In his mind he saw, in no order but in jumbled images, the Kraut dying, the soldier with the burned hand, Asch lying in the snow bleeding out of the little holes, the legs of the dead woman, the scenes of carnage going back to Salerno —

and it was all one thing, cold in him, ice at the heart, something dead as the stone where he lay. He himself was stone, a statue's eyes looking out of dead granite, sighting along the barrel of the carbine, as he knew the sniper had done. Everything he had ever been, everything he had ever believed in or hoped for, and all his memories of home — they were all gone, elsewhere, obliterated in the freezing darkness of this pass, drawing the crosshairs over the figure approaching, and feeling his own finger tightening on the trigger. He could not shoot. He let go of the trigger, brought the carbine down to his side, watching the shape come on. He experienced a tremendous urge to look upon the face, but then thought of the place where he was, this place he had come to in his life. It felt, in some wordless way, like a whole life that he had only begun to live.

He raised the carbine again, sighted, and fired.

The shot went off into the night, echoing far, and the figure dropped over, was still. Marson waited, believing that there might be others, that another figure, other figures, would come, and he would shoot whoever tried to help the one down, and he realized that he was now, himself, a sniper.

But no one came. Nothing stirred. The shape lay in the snow, perhaps a hundred yards away, quite still.

Marson did not know how long he waited. But finally he got to his feet, edged forward, running at a crouch to the next tree, keeping to the tree line. When he came level with the shape, he waited a few more minutes, then stepped toward it, feeling the wind that had risen, as if it were an opposing force. He felt that his mind had never been more clean, nor more empty. He had the sense, again without words, that life — all life, the life he had led and the life he had come to — had never been so suffused with clarity, a terrible inhuman clarity, made utterly out of precision, like the precision of gear and tackle in a machine. Except that he understood, in a sick wave, that this was utterly and only human. He walked a few paces away and retched onto the snow. He looked at the thickly darkened sky and the field and experienced an overpowering sense of this as the world, the only world. He walked back to the still form lying there in the snow. In the dark of the field, he looked at the man he had killed, and was surprised to see that it was not a German soldier but an Italian, with rope-soled shoes and a German officer's coat over him against the cold.

Probably the coat that had not been with the body of the dead officer who had served as a decoy. And this was just a bandit, a killer moving among the armies. The face was dark, thin, heavy jawed, bearded, with high cheekbones and a narrow cut of a mouth. Something lay on one of the black-whiskered cheeks, and Marson saw that it was a tooth, a molar, with its little extensions of bone. It made him sick again to see it. He moved the jaw, closed it. He took the sniper's scoped rifle away and threw it off into the snowfield. It was just him now, and the dead. Corporal Marson looked again at the open space and the tree line. This was the sniper. The rifle he had was scoped. It was the one.

He stumbled back out of the clearing and headed down to catch up with the others, moving quickly, as if running away from what he had just done. He was certain that he would not overtake them. He did not feel sick now, so much, but empty. It seemed that all the human parts of him had gone, had leeched out of him. He took a step and said his own name, and then said it again. It was just hollow sound. He knew nothing but the bitter cold and the silent woods, his own feet breaking through the crust of snow, the pain in his foot, the distant memory of a street and a house, a pregnant woman. "Do your duty," his father had said. And he could not find in his heart what the word meant anymore. Nothing meant anything. The particulars were all broken. Every single unabstract thing he thought glared at him, like an accusation. And "Do your duty" was an abstraction, and the dead made it seem ugly and irrelevant. Yet there was only the cold, and the way down, the trees bending with the weight of snow, the beautiful complications of windfall and rock and drifting that shaped the winter scene he moved through, and anyone would have said it was beautiful to see. He was alive, walking, breathing, remembering, and he had a deadness at his heart's core, a numbness, a sense of all his being having been reduced to a kind of obliterating concentration on this slow progress down the mountain.

He found Joyner and the old man and Asch not very far from where he had left them. Joyner challenged him, crouched behind a tree.

"It's me," Marson said, and felt as though he had lied. "Why haven't you gone farther than this?"

"Saul woke up and was sick. We couldn't move him," Joyner said. "I didn't want to leave you anyway, and you wouldn't either and you know it."

The old man stood there shivering, staring at Marson.

"We heard the shot," Joyner said. "I've never been so fuck'n spooked. I kept thinking what if it was you that got it."

"No."

"So you got him?"

Marson looked at the old man. "It wasn't a Jerry."

Joyner said, "What?"

"It was an Italian."

The old man said, *"Italiano?"*

"Yeah. *Italiano.*" Marson turned his carbine on the old man, who held his hands toward him.

"Un certo figlio d'una puttana fascista. Some on a bitch, Fascist."

"Somebody from your village?" Marson said.

"Collaborazionista fascista bastardo. Bastard."

"Yeah," Marson said. "Bastard."

Ridiculously, a memory came to him then of being in a high school class, at St. Anthony High School in Washington, D.C., in 1933, Sister Theresa's class in Shakespeare, and the play was *King Lear.* Students were asked to choose a passage to read aloud, and Marson had chosen the speech

201

of Edmund's that ends with the phrase "stand up for bastards." Marson had spoken the phrase with such satisfaction and such gusto that the gentle nun had taken him aside after the class to explain the problem of enjoying life's inconsistencies too much. She had used the word. He had not understood, although he knew perfectly well that she did not like the way he had said the speech.

He lowered the carbine and nodded at the old man. " 'Stand up for bastards,' " he said. He felt something of himself coming back, and it frightened him, as if his mind would not be able to support it. He did not want to think of home now, or of love, or of family, hearth, hope, or a sleep that presumed that what you left for the province of dreams would be there when you came back. He helped Joyner get Asch up onto his shoulders, and the three of them headed down again, going faster now. The way was so steep that several times they had to get down and edge along, pulling Asch with them. Marson offered to take his own turn carrying him. But Joyner refused. Asch did not utter a sound, and his breathing had grown very shallow. The clouds over the moon thickened, and the rain started again, pellets at first, tiny pieces of hail, turning to water. "Christ, no," Joyner said. "Christ Almighty no. Fuck'n *rain.*"

The snow surface, already crusted over, became slick. They could still break through it, but it was so hard now that at times they slipped on it, and the breaking through would come from falling.

They came to the last steep part of the climb, the rock ledge where they had slept a little on the way up. They settled Asch in the lee of it and got down themselves, side by side — Joyner, Marson, and the old man. Here they were again, huddled out of the rain.

"An Italian," Marson said. "I can't figure it."

"They *were* on the other side," Joyner said. "Remember?"

"I'm sick."

Joyner said nothing.

Asch stirred and moaned. He opened his eyes and stared out. For an instant, Marson thought he might be dead. "Where are we?"

"Almost there," Marson said.

"I'm dead. I can feel the blood going out of me."

"You're imagining it."

"No."

"You are. It's your imagination."

"I have no imagination anymore," Asch

said. "I'm all facts. That's me, Robert. Ask me anything." He sobbed. "Ask me if I'm gonna die."

"You'll make it. We're almost there. Save your strength. You *will* make it."

"Did you go to the serials?" Asch said. "Back home? The movie houses?"

Marson thought the other might be raving again. "Yes," he said.

"Saturday matinee," Asch said. "Remember?" He coughed — it seemed harmless, small, not connected to his wounds. He cleared his throat. "All day for a nickel."

"Yep."

"I always hated having to wait to see how it would turn out."

"Last-minute rescues," Joyner said.

"Right." Asch sobbed. "Goddamn it. I should've been in synagogue."

"Hey," Joyner said. "Marson got the son of a bitch that shot you, Saul."

"Well, then the son of a bitch and I will both be dead. *B'rikh hu.* You know what that means? That means 'Blessed is he.' "

"You'll be dead someday, like all of us," Joyner told him. "But first you're gonna be out of the fuck'n war."

"I wish I was Catholic sometimes."

"I wish I was Jewish sometimes," Marson said. He felt wrong, as if he had not taken

204

the other man seriously enough.

"I could make my confession and be happy." So it was one of Asch's jokes.

"Don't know where we'll get our hands on a priest," Marson said.

"Can't any Catholic hear it?"

"Only baptism can be done by any Catholic."

"Okay, can I be baptized?"

"Do you really want to be?"

"Might as well cover all the bases." Asch smiled. "I never believed it much. We learned the prayers. Grew up with it."

"Hey," Joyner said. "Keep still and we'll get you down this fuck'n mountain and I'll baptize you myself."

"I'm a sinner."

"We all are," said Joyner.

"You carried me, Benny." Asch was weeping again. "I'm sorry. I'm sorry, Benny."

"I'm sorry, too. You're a heavy stinking bastard."

"I am."

"You're gonna remember saying all this when you're healed up and you're gonna be embarrassed, buddy."

"I wish I could've *savored* things more."

"Well, save your breath."

After a moment, Asch choked up something and spit. He said, "Is that blood?"

They did not answer him at first.

"Fellas?"

"It's too dark to see, okay?" Joyner said.

"Is it raining *again?*"

"Like the end of the fucking world," Marson told him.

TWENTY-FOUR

Finally, they started down again, churning up the crusted snow, once more being thrashed by the rain, which was needle thin, like tiny blades of ice. Joyner, carrying Asch, fell and slid with him in the breaking-up icy melting of the snow, and Marson had to help them both move from the base of the tree that had stopped their descent. The old man was making his way down ahead of them, carrying Asch's pack.

"Saul?" Joyner said, lifting him again. "Can you see his face?" he asked Marson, who could not. "You pissed on me, Asch. Hey, Asch."

"We're almost down," Marson said.

They came at last out onto the road, where they found that a tank battalion had come up. Joyner began to try to run. "He's not breathing," he said. "Goddamn it. I think he stopped breathing." They crossed the road. Joyner set Asch down on the bed of one of the two-and-a-half-ton trucks, and a corpsman with wide, heavy wrists and sloping shoulders walked over and took Asch's pulse. He blew into the mouth and pressed the chest, and then repeated this. He hit Asch's chest three times and put the side of his head down on the breastbone. At last he straightened. "Gone," he said. He reached into the wet shirt and ripped the dog tags off, put one into Asch's mouth, and punched the chin, so that it caught between the teeth. Joyner flew at him. "You fucking stupid son of a bitch!" he said, flailing. It took two of the others to subdue him. Joyner sat weeping on the ground with his arms draped over his upraised knees, the rain splattering off his helmet and his shoulders. The others stood around watching. Marson had sunk to the ground at the wheel of a jeep that had come up. He watched two soldiers carry Asch's body away. He could not find it in himself to feel anything. It was all death. Death, death. The rain kept coming down and the others walked away from Joyner, who could not stop. Joyner's voice went off into the predawn and the rain, the rushing of the river a few yards away through the trees.

The patrol had gone on. Skirmishers had come through the trees on the other side of the river. Glick was dead. McCaig and Lockhart were casualties, already invalided out of the war.

Overnight.

A captain, tall and dark blue eyed, with wire-framed eyeglasses, walked over and looked at them. "Fuck," he said. "This whole thing's fucked. What a royal fuck up."

Angelo stood near Corporal Marson, looking guilty, almost skulking, hands tucked into the front of his cloak. He was someone awaiting release. It was evident how little any of this meant to him. Marson resented him for it. He looked for the cart and the horse, the old man's earthly goods. It was like searching for some sign of sane, livable existence.

Joyner kept shaking his head and weeping, and when the captain stood over him he looked up, his face running with the rain and his tears. "Murderers," he said.

The captain said, "Yeah. Outstanding."

"Murderers," Joyner said.

The captain turned to a couple of the others. "Get him out of here, will you?"

They took Joyner by the arms, lifting him. Marson didn't know any of them. It was as if he had left one war and come back into another.

"I'm reporting it all," Joyner said.

The others half carried, half dragged him away. The captain walked over to Corporal Marson, who stood to face him. "You wanna tell me about this?"

"He's exhausted, sir," Marson said. "He carried Private Asch most of the way down this mountain."

"You get a view of what's down the road north?"

"An orderly retreat," Marson said emptily. "A big force, moving north."

"Tell me the rest of it."

He heard himself telling about the climb, the exhaustion, the dead soldier, the sniper who was not a German skirmisher but an Italian straggler. While he told it all, Angelo stood waiting to be let go. He kept murmuring something, looking at the other soldiers, blinking in the rain.

The captain glanced at him. "Search the old man," he said to two others.

They took Angelo aside and went through his cloak. They found the little bottle of schnapps, a few coins — and a drawn map of this part of the country. The map showed positions of American units in the area. "He's a spy," the captain said. "Take him into the woods by the river and shoot him."

"What?" Marson said. *"What?"*

"You heard me."

"No, sir."

"Are you questioning me?"

"Sir — you can't mean it."

"Two soldiers in this outfit were shot by an SS officer and his whore. Four others got it last night. From Italians — acting like people happy to be liberated. You lost somebody from the same actions. Some of them are still in this, and this one's carrying around scouting information on us. I'm not taking any chances."

"He had nothing to do with this, sir."

"That's an order, Corporal. These people know the penalty for spying."

"But he helped us get where we needed to, sir. He kept his word."

"Yeah, and if they overrun us today, he'll go back to helping them scout *us*. This patrol got the shit shot out of it this morning, Corporal. They got it from a couple of peasants who looked just like him. Take care of it."

"But he isn't with them, sir. He's not with them." As Marson spoke the words he was not certain that they were true. He was not certain of anything.

"Look. You gonna do it, or will I?"

Angelo evidently realized what they were talking about. He began a low muttering and a kind of nervous dance, looking into the raining sky. *"Ave Maria,"* he said, loud, *"piena di grazia, il Signore è con te."* His voice grew still louder as the captain turned to him, and Marson realized, through the second strand of pleading words, that he was saying the Hail Mary in his native language: *"Tu sei benedetta fra le donne e benedetto . . ."*

"Sir," Marson said. "Don't do this."

The captain unholstered his pistol.

"Wait, sir," Marson said. "He's my prisoner."

The captain stopped and looked at him. Others were watching as well. The old man looked around himself, at the soldiers standing there staring at him, and he said his prayer louder, dancing in pure terror. *"Ave Maria, piena di grazia . . ."*

Marson said again, "He's my prisoner, sir."

In the next moment, the old man's bladder emptied out — the urine ran down his legs and steamed at his feet. Marson looked at the rope-soled shoes.

"Take him over into the trees and do it," the captain said. "Now."

Corporal Marson leveled his carbine at Angelo and gestured for him to move off. The old man sank to his knees, crying, folding his hands, as if Marson were an icon to which he was praying.

"Get up," Marson said, aware of the others watching him.

The old man slowly got to his feet, still with hands clasped, looking at Marson with a mixture of disbelief and fright. *"Amico,"* he pleaded. "Friend."

Marson gestured for him to walk ahead, and he began to move off in a mincing stride, weeping and saying the prayer. Corporal Marson knew the prayer well enough to repeat it with him, except that he could not recall the English. It was as if the words had never been in any other language.

They went into the trees on the river side of the road, and on down a path to the edge of the water. Marson kept gesturing for him to continue along the path, which wound away from the road. Dawn was breaking behind the heavy clouds, the sky turning to light, gray and cold, with black tatters drifting in it, and the freezing rain, still coming down, as if it had never stopped. Marson looked over his shoulder to see that he was out of sight of the road, and of the others. "Okay, hold it," he said to the old man. "Wait." Angelo stopped and turned, and now seemed to have gathered himself. There was something different about his eyes. Suddenly he said, "Pig," his mouth with its bad teeth open, his face fixed in a strange, gaping scowl.

Marson stared. The black eyes showed nothing. But then for an instant it was as if the old face had tightened with hatred.

"Santa Maria, Madre di Dio, prega per noi peccatori, adesso e nell'ora della nostra morte. Amen."

"Madre di Dio," Marson said to him.

Angelo sank to his knees. And in his face now you could see that he had nothing but loathing for the other, his expression defiant but resigned. There was an unnatural glitter of triumph in it, the look of someone who has proved himself right about something. Clearly he expected to die, and he had accepted it.

He had taken Marson and the others across the mountain because it was a way to survive, and Joyner had been right about him all along.

"Fascist," Marson said.

"Uccidami," Angelo muttered through his teeth.

"I don't understand. No *capeesh.*"

"Faccialo!"

"No *capeesh.*"

"Do! Shoot. *Ti maledico!*"

Corporal Marson raised the barrel of the carbine, leveling it at the other's middle.

"*Maledico?*" he said.

"Visit hell," Angelo said.

"You're telling me to go to hell."

"*È bene che l'ebreo è morto.*"

"I think I understand you," Marson said. He wanted to shoot now. He felt the nerve pulse travel along his wrist to his finger on the trigger.

"Is a-good the Jew die."

He aimed the rifle. "Yeah," he said. "Pig."

"*Prega per noi peccatori, adesso e nell'ora della nostra morte. Amen.*" The old man was talking fast now, eyes wide and frantic and full of hate.

Marson understood that the other had begun to pray again, and he paused once more. "You visited Washington, D.C."

"*Che cosa.*" The old man muttered the words, head bowed, trying to master himself.

"You saw New York," Marson said.

"New York, *sì.* Washington." Something like expectation showed in the eyes. "I like."

"Catholic."

"*Sì.*"

"You."

The old eyes gave back nothing. Marson stared at him, and had a moment when he thought they might begin to speak back and forth in some other language. Something

215

passed between them, a kind of silent acknowledgment of what all of this had been, and the old man was indeed Catholic. And a Fascist, too.

"Fascist," Marson said.

And then again the praying began. *"Madre di Dio . . ."*

He looked back once more in the direction of the road, then turned and let the barrel of the carbine down. *"Via,"* he said. "Just go. Get the hell away from me."

Angelo looked at him. The dark eyes were unreadable now. Water ran down the lined face. He did not move. He went on muttering the prayer.

"Get out," Marson said. "Go. Run."

"Santa Maria, Madre di Dio . . ."

"Goddamn it," Marson said, low. *"Via! Via!"*

The old man stood slowly, feebly, the legs barely holding him up, face contorted with his defiance and with the certainty that he was about to die. But then he began pleading again for his life, crying and holding out his skeletal hands. Marson felt a sudden black surge of rage, a kind of revulsion at the other's abjectness, given what he was, the pitiful shape of him there, the dark eyes pleading, and the centuries-old hatreds in him, the crying, going on, rain and tears on

216

the old face with its high twin networks of wrinkles over the eyes. Marson, in his exhaustion and his emptiness, raised the barrel of the carbine, and said, once more, *"Via."* He experienced another urge to shoot, go ahead and do it now. Do it. It would only be another Fascist. It might as well be the devil himself.

The old man turned, took a step, and then fell to his knees.

Marson walked over and put the barrel of the carbine against the base of his skull. He had been ordered to do this. The old man kept praying, and again Marson said, "Goddamn you. *Via! Via!*" He reached down and took hold of the cloak, and pulled him to his feet. Then he made a gesture, waving him away, and he fired the rifle into the wet earth. One shot. The old man jumped, and fell to the ground again, covering his face. Marson felt an overwhelming desire to be rid of him, and now he, too, was weeping. *"Via,* goddamn you. Go. Go."

At last, Angelo seemed to understand. Weeping, bowing, he got to his feet and started backing away, and he was nothing more than an old man who had tried to use both sides to go on being who he had ignorantly been all his long life. He went along the path, and around that bend of the river, still looking back, still saying the prayer. Marson sat down in the middle of the path and, laying the rifle across his knees, put his hands to his face. "Hail Mary," he said, "full of Grace. The Lord is with thee." But he could not find the rest of the words.

He wept a little, thinking of what he had come near to doing, and of what he had already done, and thinking, too, of Asch and the others. Asch was dead. And Glick was dead, too. The war had got him. There was nothing to report, now, nothing to say or do about all that. He looked where the old man had gone. Angelo, the Fascist, had survived the night. Angelo would say or be anything to survive. He was an old man in a war, on the losing side. And Robert Marson had let him go. There was not much a seventy-year-old Italian man would be able to do to change the war. And maybe something or someone else would kill him, but Robert Marson of 1236 Kearney Street in Washington, D.C., had not done so.

Morning had come, light spreading across the low sky. The corporal got to his feet and started back toward the road. Just before he reached sight of it, and the others, he stopped, feeling something rise in him. The rain was increasing. The wind had died. The clouds were showing places where sun might come through, or it might not. There was no sound of firing, and the river ran with its steady roar. He waited, breathing slowly.

It was peace. It was the world itself, water rushing near the lip of the bank from the storms, the snow and the winter rain. He felt almost good, here. He thought of home, and he could see it, that street, those people. He had found a way back to imagining it. For a few moments, he believed that he might simply stay here by this river. He wanted to. It came to him that he had never wanted anything so much. It would be perfectly simple. He would lie down and let the war go on without him, and when it was over and the killings had stopped, he would get up and go home. He thought of going off in the direction the old man had taken, of finding someplace away. Someplace far.

He turned in a small circle and looked at the grass, the rocks, the river, the raining sky with its ragged and torn places, the shining bark of the wet trees all around. He could not think of any prayers now. But every movement felt like a kind of adoration.

Then the feeling dissolved, was gone, like a breath.

His foot hurt. It was probably infected. He turned his face up into the rain and sobbed, once, like a gasp, and then it was as if he were letting go a silent scream, standing there shaking, frozen in the attitude of the scream, head turned to the sky, mouth open. No sound came. There was just the tremor, the tensed muscles, the eyes shut tight, the mouth open. The rain hit his face, and when the muscles of his jaw relaxed, he kept his mouth wide, and drank. He could not believe how thirsty he had become. He let his mouth fill with the rain, then swallowed. It was so cold. He let it fill, and swallowed again. He took one more look around himself. A pattern of the water had formed in a wild tangle of a thicket, a silver shimmer dropping onto the mud of the path. The water was so clear and clean.

He shouldered his carbine and made his way back into the war.

ABOUT THE AUTHOR

This is **Richard Bausch's** eleventh novel. He is also the author of seven volumes of short stories. His work has appeared in *The New Yorker, The Atlantic Monthly, Esquire, Playboy, GQ, Harper's Magazine,* and other publications and has been featured in numerous best-of collections, including O. Henry Prize Stories, *Best American Short Stories,* and *New Stories from the South.* In 2004 he won the PEN/Malamud Award for Short Fiction. He is Chancellor of the Fellowship of Southern Writers and lives in Memphis, Tennessee, where he is Moss Chair of Excellence in the Writer's Workshop of the University of Memphis.

The employees of Thorndike Press hope you have enjoyed this Large Print book. All our Thorndike and Wheeler Large Print titles are designed for easy reading, and all our books are made to last. Other Thorndike Press Large Print books are available at your library, through selected bookstores, or directly from us.

For information about titles, please call:
(800) 223-1244

or visit our Web site at:
http://gale.cengage.com/thorndike

To share your comments, please write:
Publisher
Thorndike Press
295 Kennedy Memorial Drive
Waterville, ME 04901

CLEVELAND PUBLIC LIBRARY
LITERATURE DEPT.

JAN 1 4 2009